Bioidentical Hormones Made Easy!

Turn back the aging clock by learning how to restore your hormones to youthful levels.

Prevent cancer, heart disease, mental decline, and other diseases of aging by avoiding the hormonal deficiency of menopause and andropause.

Look great!
Feel great!
Lose weight!
Have better sex!

Y.L. Wright, M.A.
LULU.COM

Published by Lulu.com in the United States

ISBN 978-1-257-80569-3

Printed in the United States of America

MEDICAL DISCLAIMER:
The following text is for general information only. It contains the opinions and ideas of the author. Careful attention has been paid to insure the accuracy of the information, but the author and the publisher cannot assume responsibility for the validity or consequences of its use. The intention of this book is to provide helpful information. This information is not intended to diagnose or treat any disease. This book is sold with the understanding that the author and publisher are not rendering medical, health, or any other professional services. See your medical or health professional concerning any health concerns or before following any suggestions made in this book or drawing inferences from it. The author and publisher specifically disclaim all responsibility for any liability, loss, or risk incurred as a direct or indirect consequence of using this book's contents. Any use of the information found in this book is the sole responsibility of the reader. Any dietary, nutrient, hormone, and medication suggestions found in this book are to be followed only under the supervision of a medical doctor or other endocrine specialist. Any reference to particular companies or supplements is only for the benefit of the reader. The author receives no compensation from endorsement of any product.

ACKNOWLEDGMENTS:
This book is written for you. If even one person finds their way out of chronic disease and suffering into health, it has been worth it.

ON THE COVER:
Pictured are syringes of estradiol (green) and progesterone (purple) transdermal creams.

Table of Contents

Introduction

READ THIS BOOK and CHANGE YOUR LIFE.

Develop an action plan to feel *better* as you age. Understand your hormones and immediately take easy steps to return to optimal health. Lower your health care costs. Reduce your risk of getting cancer and heart disease. See how stress depletes your hormones and what to do about it. Discover the secrets about why it is so difficult for women, but not men, to get bioidentical hormones. Find a doctor who *will* get you the bioidentical hormones that will help you and not hurt you.

Review the history of HRT (hormone replacement therapy). Explore the major research and progression of available treatments for menopause. See how irrational fear developed around the use of *all* HRT. Learn how our options have improved dramatically from our mothers' generation to ours with the availability of safe and beneficial bioidentical hormone replacement therapy (BHRT).

Understand the hormones of a healthy young woman and see how they deteriorate in perimenopause (in the years leading up to menopause) and in menopause (when the menstrual periods have ceased). Learn how to balance your hormones at any age. Recognize what happens to the hormones of men as they reach andropause (male menopause) and learn how to reverse their decline, too.

Learn about estrogen and progesterone. Understand how these hormones change as we age, when and how to use them, and how to keep levels high enough and balanced. Discover how to reduce your chances of getting cancer by removing the conditions that *cause* cancer.

Compare the ways to dose estrogen and progesterone. When used in the same dose each day, bioidentical hormones cannot be utilized well. Instead, learn how transdermal creams can be applied in levels and amounts that fluctuate throughout the month to simulate the hormonal status and good health of a young, vital woman.

See how testosterone can improve the health of both men and women. Learn how to remove toxicity, improve your diet and sleep, improve estrogen metabolism, and balance your hormones.

Master the secrets of how to look great, feel great, lose weight, and have better sex!

1: I Tried to Help My Mother

LET'S LOOK FIRST AT A WOMAN WHO ENTERED MENOPAUSE IN 1959. My mother hit menopause at age 42. I was just seven years old. I watched her physical and mental deterioration for most of my life. Let's see how it progressed from my standpoint.

I was an avid reader. By the time I got to high school, I had mentally devoured a good-sized chunk of our local library in Pennsylvania. One fine day in the late 60's I was snooping through the biology section and discovered hormones.

Because my mother was having menopausal problems, I decided to immerse myself in this fascinating subject right then and there. I needed some expert advice to figure out how to help her.

It wasn't just the hot flashes. First Mom broke her ankle and then her leg as her bones lost their density and strength (osteoporosis). I had to assume most of the household chores while she recovered. Even after she could walk again, I continued to do most of the work around the house because it was too much for her "nerves."

Her moods were volatile. She would rail at me for the slightest infraction. I escaped to the YMCA pool or my bedroom in avoidance.

Mom was depressed. She stopped working and became a permanent fixture in her Lazy Boy recliner, complaining of utter exhaustion. Then she lay wide-awake in bed at night. Her hair was falling out by the handfuls. She looked awful. She seemed to go from middle age to old age overnight. I was really concerned.

At that time there were really only two choices for a menopausal woman to deal with her fate.

The first was to do nothing but buck up and face the fact that you were getting old. You were washed up. You had lived the good life and now it was over.

After reading every hormone book in the library, I came to the conclusion that there was a good second choice. Estrogen had been proven to prevent heart disease, as well as reverse all of the nasty menopausal symptoms that I was seeing in my mother. I encouraged her to take it. Her response was, "No. It gives you cancer."

Year after year I watched the deterioration continue. I went away to college, first in Florida, and eventually on to California, New Mexico, Arizona, and Colorado. Each time I came home for vacations, aging had impacted her more brutally, but she refused to take the estrogen.

Meanwhile, I immersed myself in the study of the intricacies of the human body, primarily focusing on anatomy, physiology, and health. I got a B.A., an M.A., worked on my Ph.D., got married, had two children, and got a teaching degree. I coached swimming and taught Physical Education at the college level, the high school level, and finally K-2. After divorcing and getting married again, I re-trained in manual medicine (physical therapy of all kinds) and began to assist Joe Swartz, M.D., in his medical practice in Boulder, Colorado.

During this time, Mom suffered "mini-strokes" (blocked arteries or blood leakage in the brain), falling on her face and injuring herself badly. Her memory was fading away. My older retired siblings each took turns caring for her in their homes as her health continued to fail.

One early morning, when Mom was staying with my sister in Maine, the neighbors found our mother wandering around the streets naked, raving that her uncle (who had died decades ago) was trying to hurt her. Fortunately, these neighbors recognized her and brought her back to my sister's house.

My sister and her husband, who were just getting up, were shocked senseless. They knew that Mom was having a few mental problems, but now the situation had grown dire. The time had come for her to be put into a place where she would be safe and well-cared for. She was just 75 years old. But the aging process had taken its toll.

She went into assisted living. It was a nice place, with doors that locked to keep the residents inside. But it wasn't home.

Mom was heartbroken and complained bitterly. She constantly pleaded with us to take her home. But it wasn't safe for her at home.

She graduated to a nursing home with constant care. Every time I went back to Pennsylvania to visit, she seemed more stooped over, more confused, and angrier. Her teeth broke off and her bone density decreased. She progressed from a walker to a wheelchair. One day while they were moving her, her ankle broke. Her bones had weakened so much that they could not support her own weight. She never walked again. She became so weak that she could do nothing for herself. She couldn't feed herself, get up to go to the bathroom, or even lift her head to look at you.

Now, at 93, my mother does not know who I am. Her mental faculties have completely vanished. I wish that she could understand me when I tell her that I love her.

2: The Third Choice

WE NOW HAVE A THIRD CHOICE. We don't have to suffer a similar fate. When menopause began its dreadful attack on my mother's health, the only two choices were to do nothing, or to go to the doctor and get Premarin (horse estrogen).

We can choose bioidentical hormones. We are so lucky. We don't have to choose between no hormones or dangerous hormones that were created in a laboratory. We now can choose bioidentical hormones. These bioidentical hormones exactly match those made by the human body. As the shapes of these hormones are identical to our own hormones, they do not cause the serious health problems caused by the artificial hormones made by the pharmaceutical companies. In fact, these bioidentical hormones, when used properly, can *prevent* the heart disease, cancer, mental decline, and health problems common to menopausal women.

Our bodies recognize bioidentical hormones as safe and are able to break them down easily. We can use them effectively and easily get rid of the by-products. Many studies offer evidence that bioidentical estrogen and progesterone are quite safe with positive effects on bone, brain, breasts (the 3B's), heart, and other organs.[1] [2] [3]

But Premarin is still used by millions of women all over the world to deal with their menopausal symptoms. If you go to your family doctor today, there is a good chance that you will be given Premarin to treat the symptoms of menopause. You may get anti-depressants, some meds to control your cholesterol, and perhaps some thyroid meds as well. You may get Provera, (fake progesterone) which has been proven to cause heart disease, cancer, and gall bladder problems. The deadly cocktail of drugs may help for a little while, but eventually it will cause more problems than it ever helped.

Premarin and Provera are dangerous drugs. They are identified as foreign by our bodies, cannot be used effectively, and damage our cells. When drugs are broken down, by-products are formed. These by-products are often even more powerful than the original drug. They build up and build up, drastically increasing cancer risk and other side effects. Women who use synthetic hormones like Premarin, Provera, and the combination, PremPro have a much greater risk for breast cancer and heart disease (which kills many more women than breast cancer). Let's see now why *all* hormones have come to be feared, even if they are bioidentical. Let's look at the recent history of HRT.

3: A Little Hormone History

LET'S SEE HOW WE GOT WHERE WE ARE.

Looking at the history of HRT will allow you to understand the current political climate in the medical world and see why most doctors won't prescribe BHRT.

The drug companies can't make money selling natural substances. You can't get a patent on a natural substance, only on an invented drug. The way drug companies make money is to take a natural substance and change it into a drug. Then they can get a patent on their drug. When they have a patent, they can charge whatever they want for their drug. The drug companies then make money . . . *lots* of money.

The artificial hormones that they make act sort of like our own hormones and do relieve the symptoms of menopause. But these drugs have side effects . . . like *death*.

Research has mostly focused on Premarin, because the drug companies pay for the research.

Research showed that Premarin reduces heart disease, diabetes, and overweight. An important study published in 1991 studied 48,470 post-menopausal women for ten years.[4] They found a significant reduction in heart disease and death from heart disease in women who used what they called "estrogen," but was actually Premarin. These Premarin users also were less likely to be overweight or to develop diabetes.

A study published in 1992[5] compiled the results of *all* of the English language hormone studies done since 1970. All of this research showed that deaths as a result of heart problems were only half as likely in women who were taking hormones, even if they were synthetic. So far, Premarin was looking pretty good.

Doctors began prescribing Premarin like crazy. Premarin was usually prescribed alone.

But Premarin builds up the lining of the uterus and causes cancer. The toxic by-products of this altered horse hormone are very powerful foreign hormones that still stimulate human tissue. Without some form of progesterone, the lining of the uterus of a woman taking Premarin will build up and build up, without being shed as a menstrual period. This frequently causes the inside of her uterus to become cancerous. From 1993-1998, studies found that women who took Premarin without progesterone (unopposed estrogen) eventually got endometrial cancer.[6] [7] [8] [9] [10] The drug companies had to figure out how to stop the endometrial cancer caused by Premarin.

Bioidentical progesterone solved that problem.
Researchers then discovered that real, bioidentical progesterone would prevent cancer.[11] [12] The real progesterone was added for two weeks out of the month to simulate a woman's normal rhythm.

But the drug companies couldn't make money selling bioidentical progesterone because it was
unpatentable. The drug companies had to come up with something that acted *like* the bioidentical progesterone, but was a *drug* that they could patent, charge a lot for the drug, and then rake in the big bucks.

So they made Provera. They took real bioidentical
progesterone and altered it in the lab.

Provera was added to Premarin into a daily pill.
They called this deadly combination PremPro.

PremPro kills women. Premarin, taken alone, is
associated with increased risk of cancer of the uterus, clots in the deep veins, stroke, and dementia. PremPro is associated with increased risk of heart attack, stroke, invasive breast cancer, pulmonary emboli, and deep venous thrombosis.[13] Premarin and Provera were proven so dangerous in the largest study ever done on HRT (the Women's Health Initiative) that the entire study was halted prematurely because of the number of women dying from PremPro.

PremPro causes heart disease.[14] In 1998, at the
HERS trial,[15] researchers concluded that, "The treatment *did* increase the rate of thromboembolic events and gallbladder disease."

Did researchers stop experimenting with dangerous synthetic combinations? No! The drug
companies were desperate to prove that their synthetic drugs worked and to keep bioidentical hormones out of women's reach. So even though PremPro had been proven to cause heart disease, they went ahead and did the biggest and grandest study of them all looking at Premarin and Provera.

In 2002, the Women's Health Initiative (W.H.I.) took place to study Premarin and Provera.[16] Because
the drug companies were paying for the study, they conveniently forgot the results of the studies done four years earlier and went ahead and gave the deadly drug combo, PremPro, to their experimental subjects in their massive study using 16,608 postmenopausal women. They did not use any bioidentical hormones

at all. Just to confuse the issue, they called the Premarin "estrogen."

The results were so heinous that the study was halted long before they had planned to end it. They found that women taking Premarin and Provera (PremPro) were developing cancer and heart disease at alarming rates.[17] The researchers concluded that, "Overall health risks exceeded benefits from use of combined estrogen plus progestin." Panic ensued. Sales of PremPro tanked.

Faulty terminology caused people to believe that all HRT caused cancer and heart disease. The W.H.I. study *only* looked at women taking PremPro. This combination of horse urine estrogen and the artificial progesterone caused both heart disease and cancer. By calling Premarin "estrogen," people reading the study concluded that all estrogens were bad. Because of wrong language, people also assumed that Provera was the same as natural bioidentical progesterone.

Bioidentical hormones were dismissed as dangerous, when they never even looked at them in this study. It was confusing and unfortunate. Hormone hysteria reigned after the Women's Health Initiative was published. Women and health care providers became afraid of *all* HRT even though real, bioidentical hormones had not been tested in this study.

Fear is a powerful emotion. People focused on the fact that the combination of Premarin and artificial progesterone (PremPro) increased cancer and heart disease.

Because they didn't know the difference between synthetic and bioidentical hormones, all hormones were condemned as dangerous. This is why most doctors will not prescribe BHRT and why many women fear using any kind of HRT. They falsely believe that *all* HRT causes heart disease and cancer. This is really unfortunate, because BHRT could save women and men from the very diseases that they fear . . . if only they could see the truth. The truth is that the synthetic and horse hormones that are produced by the pharmaceutical companies are dangerous. They are produced because of greed, with absolute disregard for the health of those who use them.

Bioidentical hormones are safe and protective. If you must fear something, fear the lack of hormones that will be your fate if you *don't* supplement them bioidentically as you become hormonally-deficient.

A4M and ACAM teach physicians about bioidentical hormones and anti-aging. Fortunately, there are a few forward-thinking health professionals who can see through the confusion. The American Academy for Anti-Aging began offering seminars and educational programs to teach physicians how to prescribe BHRT in 1992. The American College for Advancement in Medicine (ACAM) was formed in 1985. They also are dedicated to training physicians about wellness and prevention of illness. The formation of A4M and ACAM were the beginning of women's chances to actually *get* BHRT.

Dr. Lee popularized bioidentical progesterone. In

1996 a retired doctor named John Lee wrote a landmark book about hormones. It was called, <u>What Your Doctor May Not Tell You about Menopause</u>.[18] He outlined how to use progesterone to help women who were losing their own progesterone in the years leading up to menopause. The progesterone that he advocated was not the artificial kind, Provera, but instead was exactly identical to the progesterone made in the female body during ovulation (when an egg is released).

Dr. Lee argued that since progesterone was the first hormone to decline as women age, it should be the first to be replaced. He used the term, "estrogen dominance" to describe the hormonal imbalance caused when progesterone drops in relation to estrogen in the decades before menopause. He encouraged doctors to prescribe natural bioidentical progesterone to restore hormonal balance to these estrogen-dominant women.

This natural, bioidentical progesterone advocated by Dr. Lee can only be obtained from compounding pharmacies. Compounding pharmacies mix their own preparations using natural substances that are tailored exactly to meet each individual's own needs.   But, although it is very helpful in perimenopause, progesterone alone can't balance women's hormones in menopause if their estrogen also becomes deficient.

T.S. Wiley rocked the hormone world. In 2003,

Wiley, along with Taguchi and Formby, published <u>Sex, Lies and Menopause</u>.[19]   Each heading of this book refers to a rock and roll song. This novel rhythmic approach was used to convey the message that if hormonal replacement is to be effective, it must mimic the rhythmic monthly hormonal surges that occur in a young woman's menstrual cycle. Wiley coined the slogan, "The Relief is in the Rhythm," to stress the importance of bringing back the rhythmic interplay of our hormones that is lost in aging.

Wiley made it easy for women to get their rhythm back. In defiance of the greedy drug companies and in

support of women's rights, Wiley developed a bioidentical hormone delivery protocol that is produced by compounding pharmacies which meet her own exacting standards. She trains doctors to use her protocol at seminars in Southern California.

Wiley is a target for competitors who attempt to defame her. Because her bioidentical hormone replacement protocol is so effective, interviewers attack her left and right. Such an effective and safe hormone treatment program is threatening to pharmaceutical HRT sales. But the smear campaign isn't working. Intelligent women flock in droves to doctors who prescribe the Wiley Protocol®.

This easy-to-implement program has allowed many women to use BHRT to bring back their own hormonal rhythms that were lost as they aged. The Wiley Protocol® is giving them back their lives by restoring their energy, sex drive, and joy in living. These women are reversing and avoiding all of the diseases of aging, especially osteoporosis, heart disease, and Alzheimer's.

We need more BHRT research. But the research we do have is very positive. Because the drug companies provide most of the funding for hormone research, studies examining bioidentical hormones are small and few. More research is needed to prove that bioidentical hormones are safe.

In 2006, Moskowitz[20] concluded that, "Bioidentical progesterone does not have a negative effect on blood lipids or vasculature as do many synthetic progestins, and may carry less risk with respect to breast cancer incidence. Studies of both bioidentical estrogens and progesterone suggest a reduced risk of blood clots compared to non-bioidentical preparations. Bioidentical hormone preparations have demonstrated effectiveness in addressing menopausal symptoms."

In 2009, Holtorf published a summary of all of the studies done which looked at the safety and efficacy of bioidentical hormones as compared to synthetic variants.[21] He concluded that, "Physiological data and clinical outcomes demonstrate that bioidentical hormones are associated with lower risks, including the risk of breast cancer and cardiovascular disease, and are more efficacious than their synthetic and animal-derived counterparts. Until evidence is found to the contrary, *bioidentical hormones remain the preferred method of HRT.*"

Ruiz did a study this year (2011) showing that BHRT improves menopausal symptoms, improving mood, decreasing irritability, anxiety, hot flashes, and night sweats.[22]

Formby and Schmidt did another study this year (2011).[23] They looked at 29 menopausal women taking the Wiley Protocol®. This consisted of natural estradiol and progesterone used transdermally and cyclically. They found symptomatic relief in 93% of these women. There were NO adverse side effects.

Now let me tell you about my own hormone story.

4: My Story

My own hormonal decline began in my thirties, just as my mother's deterioration had started in her thirties. But I didn't recognize the fact that my own hormones were declining and needed to be replaced. I guess I didn't think it would ever happen to me. I thought of myself as invincible to aging.

It started with small problems. As my bone density decreased over the years, I broke my leg, my ankle, my toe, and several ribs. My teeth were breaking off and I had to have one pulled out completely.

Then things got more serious. At age 45, my heart started to skip beats, and a cardiologist ordered me to stop exercising completely for about a year.

At the age of 47, my adrenal glands started to become exhausted. The adrenal glands are small glands that sit on top of the kidneys and secrete hormones that help you to cope with stress. At first, I could just rest for a few days and then regain the energy to go back to hard work for a few days.

But by the time I hit 50, my adrenal glands had given out completely. I had adrenal exhaustion that was so severe that I had to stop working and exercising altogether. My adrenals were toast.

This was very hard emotionally for me. My self-esteem went down the toilet. I had been a world-class athlete, and my job doing manual medicine required a lot of strength. My whole identity revolved around my physical strength and endurance. Now all I could do was rest. Even short exercise or work sessions left me bed-ridden for days.

At 51, I had my last period. A year later I was officially in menopause.

The hot flashes were the least of my worries.

My thyroid gland stopped working next. I began to take thyroid meds hoping to stop the profound fatigue, hair loss, and constipation. It helped a bit, but didn't alleviate these problems.

I got one vaginal infection after another. The antibiotics I took for these infections disrupted my intestinal flora and resulted in yeast infections. My pap smears were coming back abnormal.

In an attempt to bring my energy back at 52, I started to take Growth Hormone (long chain IGF-1). It made me feel great! But after only two weeks on the Growth Hormone, a deadly skin cancer, squamous cell carcinoma, began to grow out of the end of my nose. Four thousand dollars and a dreadful operation later, the cancer was gone. I was left with a scar on my nose as the only evidence of the ordeal. I learned the hard way not to mess around with Growth Hormone. I was lucky that this was a visible cancer. If dormant cancer cells had been in a more hidden place, the Growth Hormone could have promoted them to grow into a life-threatening illness that could have killed me before I even knew what had happened.

Some of my friends weren't so lucky. They no longer walk with us on this earth because of their use of steroids like this. I discuss safer alternatives in my last book, <u>Secrets about Bioidentical Hormones</u>.[24]

I took anti-depressants so that I could function,
but I was still depressed. My memory was becoming poorer and poorer, and I found it hard to concentrate. It became harder and harder to read books. My hair was falling out. My allergies were terrible. My hands were swelling up, and my wrists and fingers hurt. I started on Armour Thyroid, because my thyroid tests came back super low. I developed a cataract in my eye and had to have surgery to get a new lens. Worst of all, I was losing interest in sex. My husband's touch felt annoying. I felt old. I was grumpy. I was a mess.

At 55, my doctor wrote a prescription for Premarin for vaginal dryness. I threw it in the trash. I knew there had to be a better way.

I didn't want to end up like my mother. But I didn't want to get cancer, either. That's when I began my intensive study of anti-aging.

I read all of the hormone books that I could get my hands on. Most of them did not even mention bioidentical hormones. The ones that did mention bioidentical hormones did not give a complete picture. I couldn't find the detailed, objective information I needed from books. It wasn't there. In an attempt to find out how to go about replacing my lost hormones, I started going to medical conferences with anti-aging specialists, bought CD's of lectures describing all of the latest research findings, and listened to them over and over. I was grateful that I had a good background in human anatomy and physiology, because the lectures were aimed at medical doctors. I took all that welcome information from the bioidentical hormone gurus and ran with it. I began to implement what I was learning into my own health regimen.

I discovered the Wiley Protocol®. It made sense to me. I found a doctor who would prescribe it for me. At first, I started to rub the cream on the back of my arms, as directed on the instructions. I found out that it wouldn't work for me when applied that way. I have so little fat on the back of my arms from my lifetime of swimming that the cream couldn't be absorbed there. But when I put it on the inside of my upper legs where there *is* plenty of fat, the magic happened.

I rubbed the natural bioidentical estrogen and progesterone creams into the fat on the inside of my legs twice a day. The purple tubes contained the progesterone. I remembered that because purple and progesterone both start with "P." The green tubes had the magic estrogen cream that would make my life "go" again in every way. I changed the doses each day to whatever was written on my calendar according to the Wiley Protocol®.

The change in my hormones was absolutely shocking for the first few months. I went from zero hormones to full-tilt throttle. My moods were volatile. My breasts hurt. My ovaries hurt. It was like going through puberty all over again as the hormones woke up dormant tissues. But it was puberty in overdrive. I kept to myself a lot, so as not to subject others to my moods. I could have started at a half dose and gone more slowly, but then I never could do anything half-way. The smart thing to do would have been to restore the hormones gradually as they declined during my thirties and forties. But I didn't have this information then. So, once I figured out my problem and what to do about it, I went full-tilt boogie, baby. Whatever it took to heal, I was game. I knew I would get used to these hormones of my twenties and that eventually I would adjust.

My moods did even out after a few months. My mind cleared, and I weaned off of the anti-depressants that I had been taking for the last five years. My ovaries stopped hurting. My breasts gradually hurt less and less and finally stopped hurting most of the time when I began to take DIM[25] to correct my abnormal estrogen metabolism. When I am on the progesterone days, I often feel tingling in my breasts as the ducts heal. The mastitis I got while breast-feeding my youngest son left me with painful knots in my breasts. My breasts are healing with the Wiley Protocol®.

I changed my lifestyle by changing my diet. I began eating more protein, good oils, and cholesterol-containing foods. Cholesterol is essential to making hormones. Although I had been a vegetarian for 35 years, I converted to becoming a full-on meat eater, eating bacon, pork chops, steaks, buffalo, and hamburgers three times a day. I gave up being thin. I put on twenty-five pounds. My husband loved the change in menus and in me. There was more of me to love. As my metabolism healed, I lost ten of those pounds and settled at a good, healthy weight for me. I took tons of herbs and vitamins. For about a year, I took small amounts of Cortef (a prescription bioidentical hormone to replace the stress hormone that my adrenals could no longer produce).[26] But the degree of harm I had done to my adrenals was so severe that it would take many years to repair.

Lifestyle changes were the big guns. I re-prioritized my life to remove as much stress as possible. I sold our Colorado real estate and eventually moved us into a cheap rental on the beach in California. I began to sleep as long as humanly possible. It is not unusual for me to sleep 11-13 hours every night. But 9-10 hours is a must. My bedroom is totally dark, quiet, and temperature-controlled.

When I began to think better, I became more motivated to do something good for the world. Since I couldn't return to my hard physical work, I decided to write. As there wasn't a comprehensive bioidentical hormone book that really discussed all of the options available, I began to write one. I continued my research and published a popular scientific book about bioidentical hormones called <u>Secrets about Bioidentical Hormones</u>.[27] It includes treatment programs that can be used by doctors to balance all of the hormones.

The Wiley Protocol® is really working for me to heal all of my previous health issues. In the last three years, my bone density has gradually increased from a level that was not so great (-1 standard deviation) to a level that is excellent (+1 standard deviation). My thyroid is working better now. My hair is slowly growing back. My pap smears are normal. My allergies are completely gone. This is amazing, as I had hay fever every spring and summer for the last twenty years! The swelling and pain in my fingers and wrists disappeared. I sleep well at night. My energy came back, and my life came back online.

My sex life is amazing. My relationship with my husband has become much closer and deeper. I know now that I am not doomed to my mother's fate. I am feeling younger and more optimistic now. Life is very good.

If I knew then what I know now, I would have started BHRT when I was much younger, around age 35, before things really started to fall apart. I still do not have the level of energy I had in my thirties and early forties. I believe that if I had started BHRT then, I would be functioning nearer to that level.

Instead, I am making a gradual comeback. I am one of the lucky ones. I am grateful to all of the bioidentical hormone researchers who made it possible for me to get my life back. My goal is to inspire *you* and give *you* the information that *you* need to make decisions about *your* hormones that will prevent the inevitable decline that comes with aging, especially aging in this modern world.

Next, let's see why everyone is so confused about hormones.

5: Clearing Up the Confusion

DOCTORS DO NOT LEARN THE TRUTH about bioidentical hormones in medical school. Pharmaceutical substitutes are promoted. The lack of research on BHRT is used to persuade them that bioidentical hormones are not "proven" to be safer than pharmaceutical substitutes. The extensive research presented by ACAM and A4M experts is excluded.

Doctors often mistakenly use the term, "estrogen," when they prescribe Premarin, a horse estrogen made from pregnant mare's urine. They mistakenly use the term, "progesterone" to refer to various synthetic variants. The words "estrogen" and "progesterone" accurately refer only to bioidentical hormones. "Estrogen" and "progesterone" should not be used to refer to synthetic hormones or hormones from other species. Since most studies have only examined women taking synthetic hormones, most doctors are leery of using bioidentical hormones for women, because they don't understand the difference and have not studied the available BHRT research. Doctors reading studies that use the term "progesterone" when referring to progestins (artificial progesterone substitutes) conclude that progesterone is responsible for multiple health risks, when it was actually the use of synthetic progestins that caused the problems.[28]

Many people now fear cancer because it has been shown to be associated with HRT. Their fears are based on the outcomes of the use of horse hormones and synthetic hormones. Unfortunately, these fearful people do not understand that bioidentical hormones are relatively safe and offer protection against the very diseases of which they are afraid.

BHRT protects us. Heart disease kills 31% of all American white women ages 50-94. Heart attacks and strokes each kill more women than breast cancer and endometrial cancer combined. BHRT protects against heart disease, strokes, and osteoporosis. When used cyclically, BHRT also protects against cancer, especially uterine.

Perhaps the real "wisdom" of aging is shown by those who take advantage of the gift of BHRT. This gift keeps on giving to those who accept it, as they continue to live long and productive lives, free of the host of ailments and degenerative diseases that would have been their fate if they had opted to take the "natural" route. BHRT may restore libido and vitality, leading to a better, closer relationship. BHRT can preserve a happy marriage, allowing both partners to live life to its fullest.

6: Live Long *and* Healthy with BHRT

NATURE REMOVES PEOPLE WHEN THEY CAN NO LONGER REPRODUCE. Once the children are raised, non-reproductive members of the species are a waste of food that could be used for those who *can* reproduce. As the hormones necessary for reproduction disappear, we experience a decline in health of every organ system and tissue. Now medicine keeps many of us alive, even if we are diseased, crippled, and unable to think well.

Disease and accidents killed most of our ancestors when they were young. A hundred years ago, people didn't live long enough for aging to have become such an issue as it is today. The average age of death for women in 1900 was 46 years and for men 48 years. Now the average age of death for women is 81 and men 78. That's an extra 35 years for women and 30 years for men. Medical advances, like antibiotics, blood pressure meds, and surgery allow many of us to live well into our 90's or 100's.

We now live decades longer. Living longer without adequate hormones has resulted in escalating rates of Alzheimer's, osteoporosis, heart disease, cancer, hearing and eye problems, and other diseases. Most of us will live long, yet miserable lives. Although we are living longer, our lives are filled with sickness and disability.

We also face health issues unknown in the past. The toxic environment, altered food supply, artificial light, and injury from synthetic hormones in birth control pills and menopausal treatments have created health issues never faced before. That is why the numbers of U.S. women getting breast cancer have gone from one out of eighty to one out of nine and may soon be one out of four.

We can fool nature with BHRT. When we restore our hormones to youthful levels, each organ and tissue will receive the hormones necessary for health. BHRT can prevent health problems, allowing us to continue to live productive lives without becoming dependent on others in old age. You can choose to be healthy, active, and vibrant right up to the very end of your life if you replace your missing hormones with bioidentical ones. Or you can choose the "natural" route, with no replacement of deficient hormones, and increase your risk for virtually every discomfort, disease, physical, and mental disability.

7: Women Have Not Yet Achieved Equal Medical Rights!

WOMEN MUST TRY HARDER THAN MEN TO GET HELP WITH THEIR HORMONES.

What's good for the gander should be good for the goose. In the medical world, women have *not* achieved equal rights to those of men. Unlike a man, if a woman wants BHRT, (especially cyclic) she can't just go to any doctor and get it. Most doctors *won't* prescribe female BHRT.

Doctors say that andropause (male menopause) is a disease that should be treated. It is accepted medical fact that low levels of male sex hormones are associated with disease, loss of vitality, and length of life in males. When a male's sex hormones drop below normal laboratory reference values, he is considered to be "hypogonadal." The standard of care is to treat this deficiency state with supplemental hormones. This means that any physician would be negligent *not* to treat this condition *in a male*.

Doctors say that menopause is not a disease that should be treated. Unlike their view of andropause as a disease state that should be treated, most physicians view menopause as a healthy, natural state of life, to be treated temporarily, if at all, with antidepressants and synthetic hormones, usually given orally (pills).

I believe that the SAME standard of care should be used for men and women. Just as andropause is a hormone-deficient state caused by testosterone dropping to subnormal levels in men, the same standard of care should be applied to the treatment of menopause and perimenopause in women when *they* are hormone-deficient. I think that when women have subnormal sex hormone levels, the standard of care should be BHRT, just as the standard of care for men is BHRT when *their* sex hormones become subnormal.

Let's move on to looking at the hormones in a healthy young woman, how they become imbalanced as we age, and how to find a doctor who *is* willing to go out on a limb and treat our hormone deficiencies fairly, regardless of the prevailing political climate in the medical world.

8: Why *Young* Women are Healthy

LET'S SEE HOW HORMONES WORK IN A YOUNG WOMAN IN HER PRIME.

The interplay of estrogen and progesterone in varying amounts throughout the month insures her health. Estrogen increases during the beginning of the menstrual cycle, and surges to a peak on day 12 of the menstrual cycle. The estrogen thickens the lining of the uterus to prepare it for a fertilized egg. At ovulation on day 14, the empty egg sac begins to produce progesterone, which builds up to a peak on day 21. If the egg is not fertilized, hormone levels drop and the uterine lining is shed in the form of the menstrual flow.

Surges of each hormone prepare the cells to receive the other hormone. The estrogen surge prepares the cells to receive the progesterone. The progesterone surge prepares the cells to receive estrogen. A peak of each hormone is critical in order to prepare the cells to receive the other hormone.

This happens all over a young woman's body. As the estrogen builds to a peak, cells all over her body are sucking up that estrogen and building strong, healthy tissues. The estrogen surge gets the cells ready to take in the progesterone. Then the cells take in that progesterone, just as it magically appears on day 14. The progesterone destroys any cells that shouldn't be there anymore. Those old and useless cells are then carried off and eliminated. The progesterone surge on day 21 then gets the cells ready to take in estrogen and the whole cycle begins again.

This process keeps her bones strong. It prevents osteoporosis, keeping bones strong and young.

It protects her heart. Estrogen makes new healthy heart cells, which keep her heart beating strong and steady. The progesterone then comes in and removes the old cells to make way for the newer cells that will be built as it prepares the cells to take in the estrogen again.

In her brain, the process keeps her sharp. Estrogen builds the coverings of the nerve cells that transmit the signals that keep her memories sharp. Estrogen and progesterone work to renew the brain cells that keep her thinking at the top of her game. This hormonal interplay prevents mental decline, Alzheimer's, and senile dementia. The monthly estrogen surge is essential for the health of all her nerves and brain cells.[29] [30]

The estrogen surge protects her nerves all over her body by building up the protective sheath around them. The progesterone prevents irritability and depression.

The process protects her breasts. The estrogen builds healthy new breast cells and gets the cells ready to receive the progesterone. The progesterone comes into the cells and destroys any old, cancerous, unwanted cells, and takes them out to the trash. The milk ducts stay strong, healthy, and free of cancer.

The process keeps her blood vessels healthy. The estrogen builds healthy new cells in her veins and arteries and gets them ready to receive progesterone. The progesterone carries away the old, dangerous cells that might cause trouble. The progesterone gets the cells ready to receive the estrogen again. The blood vessels stay clear, preventing venous blood clotting, arterial spasms, strokes and heart attacks.

This same process happens in over 300 tissues in the body that require these monthly surges of estrogen and progesterone to keep them healthy. As long as hormone levels remain high enough and surge, the bones will be strong, health will be good, sex drive will be healthy, and mental function will be sharp.

Each month, the estrogen surge nourishes cells all over the body insuring that all of the organs remain healthy. The estrogen surge opens the cell doors welcoming progesterone to come right on in. The progesterone breaks down unwanted and useless cells and carries them away. This monthly interplay of these two important hormones insures our health by a constant building up, breaking down, and then rebirth. When we are young and healthy, we have new construction going on and old construction being torn down monthly. New cells are born and the old cells die so that new cells can be born again.

This process prevents cancer, heart disease, memory loss, arthritis, or other diseases common to aging women. Tissues all over the body, including the joints, colon, brain, breasts, ovaries, and heart must have these rhythmic surges of estrogen and then progesterone if we are to remain in good health.

This dance of building up and breaking down maintains our health . . . until the dance is over. In order for the menstrual flow to happen, there must be enough estrogen to open the cells to receive progesterone, and there must be enough progesterone for just two weeks out of the month to prepare the cells to receive estrogen. When estrogen and progesterone decline enough, the dance is over. The music stops.

9: Progesterone Declines First.

TROUBLE HAPPENS WHEN HORMONES AREN'T PRODUCED IN ADEQUATE AMOUNTS AND/OR IN SURGES. Monthly rhythm is critical for health. Let's see how we can avoid trouble as we age.

Progesterone (P4) balances estrogen. Estrogen causes you to retain water. Progesterone helps you to get rid of fluids.

Progesterone is the first hormone to decline as women age. It declines long before estrogen declines. It should be the first one to be supplemented as we age to prevent the condition of estrogen dominance, where there is too much estrogen in relation to progesterone. If that happens, we become susceptible to abnormal growths, like cancer, fibroids, and cysts. When progesterone is deficient, even low levels of estrogen in the body may lead to breast cysts, cancer and other reproductive organ cancers.

Progesterone (P4) protects women:

- **Protects the breasts and other female organs from cancer.**
- **Builds and maintains the bones.**
- **Protects the heart, blood vessels, and nerves.**
- **Helps thyroid hormone to work better.**
- **Increases the sensitivity of cells to estrogen.**
- **Increases scalp hair.**
- **Reduces insulin levels, regulates blood sugar, reducing diabetes.**
- **Is thermogenic—helps burn fat to make energy.**
- **Helps decrease blood pressure.**
- **Lowers cholesterol and raises good HDL.**
- **It calms you.**

Progesterone is effective for two reasons:

(1) Progesterone makes estrogen work better.
When taken for two weeks out of four, progesterone tells cells all over the body to get ready to allow estrogen to come in and be used. The cells hear the progesterone knocking on their doors and open up to allow the estrogen to come on in. The estrogen is then used to create

new, healthy cells all over the body.

(2) Progesterone removes old and cancerous cells.

After growth of cells stimulated by estrogen, progesterone in the last half of the cycle produces cell death. The interplay of the two hormones brings health to women. Progesterone for two weeks out of the month mimics the normal cycle of growth and destruction. This monthly cycle brings health to tissues all over the body, including the brain, bones, breast, and heart.

Tissues that are built up have to be taken down again or they will cause trouble. Estrogen builds things. Progesterone removes the garbage.

DON'T REPLACE ESTROGEN WITHOUT REPLACING PROGESTERONE

as well. If estrogen is given without progesterone, it is called "unopposed estrogen," and may lead to cancer. If your doctor wants to give you estrogen cream for vaginal dryness without giving you progesterone, this is not OK. It causes estrogen dominance and estrogen dominance is not OK.

Estrogen dominance is by far the most common hormonal problem for women at any age. Estrogen dominance underlies PCOS (polycystic ovary syndrome), FDB (fibrocystic disease of the breast), fibroids, PMS (pre-menstrual syndrome), and excessive bleeding. Estrogen dominance is caused by progesterone deficiency. The only effective treatment is bioidentical progesterone.

Use only natural, bioidentical progesterone--P4.

It has been approved by the FDA.[31] When replacing progesterone, don't use progesterone substitutes, like Provera. Remember, most doctors don't understand the difference. They often say that they are prescribing "progesterone" when they are actually referring to synthetic variations made by pharmaceutical companies. Synthetics do not have the beneficial effects of natural progesterone. Don't try to replace progesterone with creams you can buy on the internet or health food stores, either. They are not standardized and not bioidentical. You don't know what you are getting and you don't know how much you are getting (if anything). Even if they are potent concentrations, they are not bioidentical.

Bioidentical hormones are available only by prescription. Physicians are in complete control of BHRT to meet your hormonal needs. Your doctor can prescribe the exact amount you need after testing you. It can be made in just the right amount for you by a compounding pharmacy. Then you can balance your hormones exactly. Don't mess around with your health. Do it right!

Stress eats up progesterone. If a woman is under constant stress, her adrenals are always pumping out high levels of stress hormones. These hormones are made from progesterone. High levels of stress hormones may lead to a progesterone-deficient state at *any* age.

Symptoms of low progesterone include:

- Mood swings, irritability, depression, anxiety, panic attacks.
- Fatigue.
- Allergies, inflammation, immune problems, arthritis.
- Cramping.
- Acne.
- Infertility.
- Breast cysts, ovarian cysts, fibroids.
- Low libido.
- Hot flashes.
- PMS-abdominal weight gain.
- Joint pain.
- Bone loss.
- Headaches.
- Heavier bleeding (#1 cause for hysterectomy).
- Lighter sleep.
- Fuzzy thinking.

Supplementing with progesterone early enough may prevent estrogen dominance, which causes the symptoms that warrant surgical removal of a woman's uterus and ovaries.

Replacing progesterone when it is low will reduce inflammation and chronic degenerative diseases. Use it *only* on days 14-28 of the menstrual cycle to simulate normal cycles.

It is better to restore hormones to optimal levels when they are beginning to decline rather than waiting to replace them when they are largely missing and the damage has been done.

10: Perimenopause--a Dangerous Time

ANOVULATORY CYCLES ARE CYCLES WITHOUT OVULATION. Without ovulation, cycles are irregular with irregular flow.   In the decade or so before menopause, there is a period called "perimenopause" when there are months in which ovulation does not occur. If the egg is not released, progesterone cannot be released from the empty egg sac.

Thin women athletes who are training hard are often anovulatory. In some of these women, menstruation stops altogether. Poor nutrition, stress, xenoestrogens (toxins that mimic hormones), and birth control hormones also result in anovulatory cycles. PMS is caused when the egg sac doesn't produce *enough* progesterone. Xenoestrogens and estrogen dominance are the most common cause.

When progesterone drops, estrogen becomes dominant. When progesterone is not produced or is insufficient, estrogen becomes dominant because it is not balanced by progesterone. Estrogen is therefore "unopposed." We will look at estrogen dominance in detail later.

Treat estrogen dominance with progesterone. As estrogen dominance begins to occur *anytime* in the years leading up to menopause, it is a good idea to nip it in the bud by supplementing with natural bioidentical progesterone to prevent the many problems caused by estrogen dominance. *Only* on days 14-28, use a progesterone cream compounded by a compounding pharmacy. Your doctor can measure your hormones and prescribe the exact amount that you need to balance your hormones.

Don't take progesterone every day. If you do, it will eventually cause you to be unable to receive estrogen. Without estrogen, you cannot receive progesterone, either. Daily progesterone is a very bad idea.

Begin BHRT at first signs of deficiency to avoid the hormonal imbalances of the perimenopausal state, which is a dangerous time for women. Because of anovulation, estrogen becomes dominant in relation to progesterone causing women to become more susceptible to heart attacks and cancer.

By avoiding the hormonal deficiency of perimenopause, you can avoid the serious physical and mental deterioration that occurs during the initial years of hormonal decline. If there are symptoms of hormonal deficiency, your doctor should check estrogen, progesterone, and testosterone every two years until after the forties. Then these hormones should be checked every year.

Perimenopause is associated with a very different type of heart disease than that of menopause. The heart attacks women get in their forties are caused by "sudden vasospasm." The muscle in the artery tightens and won't let go. These heart attacks kill quickly, without warning. These heart attacks kill otherwise healthy young women, who are often physically fit, non-smokers.

Perimenopausal heart attacks are caused by a lack of progesterone. These perimenopausal heart attacks are more often fatal than those of menopause.

Menopausal heart attacks are caused by a lack of estrogen. Heart attacks in women who have reached menopause are caused by arteries to the heart becoming blocked with plaque. Menopausal heart attacks are the same kind that men get. Estrogen protects women from this kind of heart attack.

In perimenopause existing cancers may grow without being checked by the protective progesterone. Without progesterone, estrogen never gets turned off. As progesterone disappears, cancer can grow unchecked.

When progesterone is gone and estrogen is high, as it is in perimenopause, it sets you up to form pre-cancerous breast lesions in your breasts. This eventually may lead to breast cancer if you don't do something about it.

Unopposed estrogen causes estrogen dominance--PMS, growth of uterine fibroids, endometrial cancer, and fibrocystic disease of the breast. If the problem of progesterone absence is not addressed, estrogen dominance can get out of control.

Irregular cycles. Dropping levels of progesterone result in irregular menstruation. As perimenopause progresses, more anovulatory cycles occur. This results in irregular cycles with irregular amount and duration of flow. Prolonged periods of anovulatory cycles initially produce irregular periods with light flow. This progresses to marked thickening of the uterine lining which results in very heavy, prolonged periods. This is the most common reason for a hysterectomy. It could be avoided if BHRT begins at the first signs of deficient hormones.

Let's look at the other important women's sex hormone, estrogen.

11: Estrogen and Menopause

WHAT IS ESTROGEN? Estrogen is the hormone that causes breast development and makes women attractive to men.

Estrogen makes a woman receptive to sex. It promotes soft skin and insures the health of all the female sex organs, including the vagina. It improves senses of taste and smell, decreases appetite, improves thinking, and stabilizes mood. It is a mild antidepressant. When you have enough estrogen, it helps to protect you against schizophrenia and Alzheimer's disease. It keeps your skin thick and tight and prevents wrinkles.

Most importantly, it prevents osteoporosis and heart disease. It prevents every one of the symptoms of menopause listed below.

---

300 different tissues in males and females depend on estrogen to function well, especially the brain, the liver, the bones, the uterus, the bladder, the breast, the skin, and the blood vessels. As all of the sex hormones drop radically in menopause, BHRT can benefit quality and length of life dramatically.

Menopause happens when we lose our hormones, specifically progesterone, estrogen, testosterone, DHEA, oxytocin, and various other hormones. When our periods stop, we lose an important way to cleanse our bodies.

When a woman goes into menopause, her ovaries produce less and less estrogen until she finally starts having hot flashes. At times, she may begin to sweat and feel very hot, even though the room temperature is normal. Hot flashes and sweating at night are often the first symptoms that bring a woman's attention to the fact that she is entering menopause. This is the time when many women start to think about replacing hormones so that they can feel better. They want to feel more like their old selves again.

Hot flashes and night sweats herald menopause. Around age 45-50, the ovaries run out of eggs. Estrogen levels eventually fall below levels needed to thicken the lining of the uterus. The menstrual flow becomes lighter and more irregular and finally stops. The brain goes into overdrive in a futile effort to stimulate ovulation. The brain center that controls overheating is stimulated by this activity and causes sweating. The brain cannot shut off this activity without estrogen or progesterone. Other control centers in the brain also go haywire causing moodiness, tiredness, and temperature swings from being too cold to being too hot.

In menopause, usually both estrogen and progesterone are very low. The immune system is especially affected when these hormones drop. Without estrogen and progesterone, the immune system becomes unbalanced. It attacks the body's own tissues. When it attacks the cartilage, we get arthritis. If it attacks the thyroid, we get Hashimoto's, and the thyroid goes haywire, wrecking our metabolism. Without estrogen and progesterone, it is difficult to sleep. If you don't sleep, you frequently become insulin-resistant and gain weight.

If a woman allows a doctor to remove her uterus and/or ovaries, menopause will occur much earlier. Instead of the gradual development in natural menopause, it will happen overnight. One-third of the women in the U.S. under age 60 have had a hysterectomy. Surgeons often remove the uterus and ovaries while a woman is in her 40's for unpleasant symptoms of excessive bleeding or fibroid tumor without any serious pathology being present.

When the uterus only is removed, the ovaries will soon stop functioning, so they are often removed along with the uterus. Some surgeons remove the ovaries to prevent cancer. When the uterus is removed, symptoms include irritability, nervousness, sleeplessness, aching bones, joints, or muscles, headaches, palpitations, depression, anxiousness, vertigo, and discomfort during intercourse. The depression that results from hysterectomy is much more severe than that of natural menopause. Some women lose their sex drive completely after their ovaries are removed. Osteopenia (when bone begins to demineralize) occurs in most women two to four years after removal of the uterus and ovaries if there is no hormonal replacement.[32]

Symptoms of menopause:

- ***Getting fatter.*** As the ovaries stop producing estrogen, the body may get fatter, especially the belly, to compensate for the lost estrogen. A weak estrogen is made in the fat. The menopausal woman loses energy and doesn't feel like exercising.

- ***Difficulty sleeping.*** She will have difficulty going to sleep and often will wake in the middle of the night.

- ***Growth of facial hair and loss of scalp hair.***

- **Sexual problems** include loss of interest in sex, dislike of sex, vaginal dryness, painful intercourse, loss of clitoral sensation, loss of urine, and a decrease in orgasms.

- **Touch avoidance.** There is a slight numbness throughout the skin. The desire to touch and to be touched may disappear. Skin is dry and itchy. Being touched doesn't feel good.

- **The vagina loses tone, shrinks, thins, dries up, and hurts.** Cracks in the vaginal walls and changes in vaginal secretions encourage germs to grow.   Itching and infections occur.

- **Vulval changes.** The tissues of the vulva lose fat and moisture and may begin to bleed when bathing, towel drying, or having gentle sex. Itching causes scratching which causes bleeding. Small scars around the lips may glue the folds together.

- **Prolapsed uterus and/or bladder.** Connective tissue weakens. The uterus may drop down through the vagina and the bladder may drop through the front vaginal wall.

- **Bladder infections, increased need to urinate, and stress incontinence.** Sneezing, coughing, laughing, and dancing may cause urine to leak out of the bladder. Women may get up several times at night to urinate and wear pads in the daytime.

- **Wrinkles** form as collagen is lost.

- **Loss of height** results when discs in the spine dehydrate and connective tissue that holds you upright weakens. Osteoporosis may lead to small breaks in the bones of the spine.

- **Dizziness, palpitations, irritability, memory loss, anxiety, depression, headaches.** The heart is weakened and becomes susceptible to irregular beats. Depression is common.[33] Memory loss and other cognitive deficits occur.

12: Adding Estrogen

THINNER WOMEN HAVE LESS ESTROGEN,

as a rule. Chronic dieters, anorexics, and over-trained women athletes often have low estrogen levels. When women enter menopause, their estrogen levels drop and they may become estrogen-deficient.

Estrogen deficiency can be corrected by eating cholesterol-containing foods (butter, shrimp, organic meats), sufficient calories to maintain a healthy level of body fat, *and* taking supplemental bioidentical estrogen and progesterone.

Premarin. If you go to a traditional medical doctor and tell him that you are suffering from any of the symptoms of menopause, he may write out a prescription for Premarin. Premarin is made from the urine of a pregnant mare. Yes, a pregnant HORSE! Premarin *will* act in the human body to relieve menopause symptoms. But it is very dangerous, because the byproducts are foreign and are very hormonally active. It causes many problems, including blood clots in the legs and cancer. All of the bad things you have heard about taking estrogen came from taking Premarin or synthetic hormones that are not shaped like those produced in the human body.

Don't take Premarin or synthetic hormones. Period. End of story. This is why you need to find a doctor who is not traditional, one who is willing to prescribe bioidentical hormones, hormones that are shaped exactly like the ones produced in our bodies.

There are three bioidentical estrogens, named E1, E2, and E3, for short. They each have different properties, actions, and levels depending on age.

E1. The first is E1, or estrone. It ends in "one." E1 is a weak estrogen that causes weight gain and lowered vitality. It increases belly fat. The body makes more of it in **menopause.**

E2. The second is E2, estradiol. It contains "di," which means "two." **Estradiol is the most active and powerful estrogen. This is the most important estrogen and the one you want to replace.** It is FDA-approved.[34] This is the estrogen of your reproductive years.

E3. The third is E3, or estriol. It contains "tri" which means "three." Increased estriol is made during **pregnancy**. Data is conflicting about any protective effect against breast cancer.[35] [36] [37] [38] [39] **It may have cancer-promoting effects** because E3 is broken down into a by-product that may lead to cancer.[40] It is not FDA-approved.

Choices for Adding Bioidentical Estrogen

"Bi-Est" is a prescription usually consisting of 80% E3 and 20% E2. It comes in a gel or a cream. Because some physicians consider E3 to be the "good" estrogen, they prescribe "Bi-Est." But a harmful by-product of E3 may increase cancer risk.[41] [42]

"Tri-Est" usually consists of 80% E3, 10% E2, and 10% E1. This used to be used more frequently, but not anymore. Most experts agree that E3 is not a hormone you want to increase. Menopausal women already have too much E1. They don't need any more.

Phytoestrogens are chemicals found in plants that can act like estrogen. But when soy and other plant estrogens are used alone, without BHRT, they may ease the symptoms but do nothing to decrease estrogen dominance and restore a normal estrogen-progesterone balance.

Be careful if you are trying to correct hormonal imbalance by using phytoestrogens. Research has found that genistein (a phytoestrogen derived from soy) may cause thyroid problems.[43] [44] Your thyroid is a gland that keeps you feeling energetic and unconstipated. Resveratrol is a phytoestrogen that is *good* for your weight, bones, and mitochondrial function. It protects your nerves.[45]

When taking BHRT, using phytoestrogens may be counterproductive, as they compete with BHRT to enter the cells and increase estrogen dominance.

E2 is the best choice for estrogen replacement.

Estradiol has about 400 functions that are important to maintaining good health. When menopausal women begin to use E2, their hunger becomes regulated, and fat shifts from the belly to the hips. E2 may have a protective effect against Alzheimer's, autoimmune diseases, cardiovascular diseases,[46] and osteoporosis.[47] Estradiol stabilizes emotions. Estradiol can be taken several ways:

1. **Oral estrogens (pills) should never be used.** They are broken down into cancer-promoting by-products. You have to use two to five times more estrogen orally compared to transdermal preparations. The by-products increase body fat, triglycerides, raise blood pressure, insulin resistance, blood clots, gallbladder disease, inflammation, and increase cancer risk.[48] [49]

2. **Patches** may contain harmful chemicals and don't absorb evenly.

3. **Creams or gels** are the best way to use estrogen, as they are absorbed into the fat base and slowly released into the bloodstream, simulating how your ovaries released estrogen when you were younger. They are easy to use, are safest, and the most effective.

13: Balancing the Hormones

KEEP THE HORMONES BALANCED. If estrogen becomes too high in relation to progesterone, a state of "estrogen dominance" occurs. If you are cycling, your doctor should direct you to get estradiol measured on day 12 and progesterone on day 21 of the menstrual cycle to make sure that E2 is peaking on day 12 and P4 is peaking on day 21. It is important to maintain sufficient levels of each hormone. But even more important is to keep them balanced in relationship to each other.

ESTROGEN DOMINANCE occurs when the sum of all the body's estrogens is too high in relation to progesterone.

The most common pre-menopausal problem is estrogen excess and progesterone deficiency. You get fatigue and weight gain. Allergies may worsen. Blood clots more easily which may set you up for a stroke or embolism. Gallbladder problems develop. This estrogen-dominant state is often made worse by lack of exercise, poor diet and lifestyle choices, use of birth control pills, and toxicity caused by environmental toxins that are being taken in and stored in the body. As the years go by, the estrogen-dominant state and its symptoms worsen.

Premarin causes estrogen dominance. Premarin is particularly harmful because it is not a human hormone and cannot be broken down properly by the human body. The by-products of this foreign, non-human hormone are not easily removed from the body. Even though Premarin has been proven to be harmful, it is still being used by millions of women all over the world.

Obesity causes estrogen dominance. The fat cells produce estrogen. The majority of overweight people have hormone imbalances. They often have too much estrogen, too much insulin, and an underactive thyroid. They will not be able to lose fat until their hormones have been adjusted.

Treatment of estrogen dominance. Optimize hormones, reduce toxicity, correct abnormal estrogen metabolism,[50] reduce stress, exercise regularly, and change unhealthy dietary habits. Take fiber with the highest-fat meal of the day to eliminate excess estrogen and toxicity. Adding two to four grams of fish oil per day to the diet is helpful to lower inflammation.

Bioidentical progesterone is the treatment for estrogen-dominant women. It is important to find a physician who really understands women's hormones, knows when and how to check hormone levels, and is not afraid to prescribe BHRT.

Calcium D-Glucarate corrects estrogen excess in both men and women.[51] Because of all the xenoestrogens coming in from environmental pollutants like plastic, cosmetics, insecticides, and pesticides, most people have a huge toxic load of chemical hormones circulating in the body and there's no way for the body to get rid of them. Calcium D-Glucarate helps the body to eliminate a lot of these synthetic hormones, carcinogens, and tumor-promoters. Women who are trying to get pregnant may get pregnant after using it for a few months. It gets rid of excess estrogen quickly. Make sure to use enough. Be careful, it *may* interfere with some prescription antidepressants. You can get it in the health food store.

Symptoms of estrogen dominance include:
- Irritability, mood swings, anxiety.
- Salt and fluid retention.
- Blood clotting.
- Allergic reaction.
- Food cravings.
- Hot flashes.
- Irregular periods.
- Depression.
- Water retention, bloating.
- Sleep disturbance.
- Headaches.
- Short term memory loss.
- Craving for sweets.
- Uterine fibroids.
- Breast pain.
- Breast swelling (all month long).
- Cysts in breasts and ovaries.
- PMS.
- Breast, uterine, ovarian cancer.
- Endometriosis.
- Increased cholesterol and triglyceride levels.
- Weight gain and exhaustion.

14: Which BHRT is Best for You?

CONTINUOUS DOSING IS TAKING THE SAME DOSE EVERY DAY. It is the standard of care for those physicians who *do* prescribe BHRT, even those who are "holistic." Most physicians who are willing to prescribe bioidentical hormones will only do it in a continuous dosing method. These physicians will prescribe a small dose of estrogen cream or gel to be rubbed into the skin in the same amount every day.

They may prescribe the progesterone cream or gel to be rubbed into the skin in the same amount every day of the month. *Or* they may prescribe the progesterone cream or gel to be rubbed into the skin in the same amount for two weeks out of four. Four days at the end of the month may be designated as "hormone-free" days when no hormones are applied. With continuous BHRT, the physician's goal is to *avoid* menstrual bleeding in the menopausal woman.

CYCLIC DOSING IS CHANGING THE DOSE OF HORMONES THROUGHOUT THE MONTH TO MIMIC A WOMAN'S NORMAL CYCLE. The Wiley Protocol® is the predominant method of cyclic dosing. Menstrual periods do occur.

CONTINUOUS DOSING IS NOT THE BEST CHOICE FOR MANY WOMEN. Doctors who prescribe estrogen and progesterone to be used continuously assume that the average American woman does not want to be bothered with menstruation. Although this *is* true, if American women really understood the benefits of cyclic dosing with the resulting menstrual flow, perhaps they might change their minds.

American women don't understand how menstruation maintains their health. American females are brought up to believe that the menstrual flow is a curse.

But other cultures honor the menstrual cycle. Ceremonies are held at the moon time. The red tent is an honored celebration of feminine power.

If health is your main priority, set aside counterproductive ingrained cultural beliefs. The menstrual flow is a healthy thing. It is a time to allow toxins to leave your body.

Continuous BHRT therapy prevents osteoporosis[52] and heart disease.[53] But cyclic BHRT dosing has *additional* health advantages over continuous BHRT because it *does* imitate how a young woman's hormones change with the moon throughout the month, just as the ocean tides go high and low in response to the cycles of the moon. The moon cycle of a young woman produces a waxing and waning of hormones in her body.

> **This ebb and flow of hormones each month protects us from cancer and provides an important detoxification pathway in the form of the menstrual flow.**

Growing numbers of women are now demanding the "Wiley Protocol®." This prescription consists of the application of twice-daily creams that deliver an increasing dose of bioidentical estradiol throughout the first half of the cycle, dropping the estradiol at mid-cycle, and then continuing the estradiol at a moderate dose through the rest of the cycle. Bioidentical progesterone is added at mid-cycle, increased in dosage, and then decreased at the end of the cycle.

The Wiley Protocol® simulates the varying hormones of a healthy young woman and brings with it the monthly menstrual flow. Proponents claim that it restores their youth and health and lowers their risk of all diseases associated with aging, including heart disease, stroke, cancer, and Alzheimer's.

Few physicians will prescribe the protocol, especially those in conservative states, where malpractice insurance will not cover them if they prescribe it. To learn more and find one of the few physicians who *will* prescribe the Wiley Protocol®, get on the internet and go to www.thewileyprotocol.com.[54]

In Lights Out, Wiley describes how life evolved under the influence of fluctuating periods of light and dark.[55] The menstrual cycle is governed by the fluctuating light and dark of the moon in lunar cycles. The Wiley Protocol® works with the lunar cycle by using the new moon as day one of the menstrual cycle.

In <u>Sex, Lies and Menopause</u>, Wiley stresses the importance of imitating the natural rhythm of the hormones in a healthy, youthful female menstrual cycle in order to restore and protect our health.[56]

This process requires peaking levels of both estradiol and progesterone to work properly. The Wiley Protocol® exactly copies the changing levels of estrogen and progesterone throughout the month, with the youthful estradiol surge at day 12 and the progesterone surge at day 21. This interplay of hormonal surges helps you to balance and use these hormones.[57] [58]

Critics of the Wiley Protocol® often use the argument that too much estrogen is being prescribed. These people are operating under that fear motivation, the false assumption that all HRT causes cancer. Many still believe that *all* forms of estrogen cause cancer, and the more you take, and the longer you take it, the more likely you are to get cancer. The reality is that if you don't take enough estrogen, you won't get a menstrual period and its health benefits, including prevention of cancer.

Cyclic BHRT Prevents Cancer. On day 21 of cyclic BHRT, progesterone floods into cells all over the body that have been prepared to receive it by the estrogen surge. The progesterone increases to a peak on day 21 and prevents cancer.[59] [60] [61] [62] The progesterone surge leads to cell death in the brain, breast, uterus, and throughout the body as the body renews itself. Old and unwanted cells that could have caused cancer are carried out of the body along with the menstrual flow.

In continuous hormone replacement, not enough estrogen is given to open the cells to progesterone.[63] Without being opened enough for progesterone to do its job, old and unwanted cells cannot be carried away. If these cells cannot be removed, they are under a continuous influence to proliferate and may become cancerous. The milk ducts in the breast are especially cleaned out and healed by progesterone. Progesterone's cleansing effect protects the breast and other tissues from cancer.

Your period is your insurance against getting cancer. A regular monthly flow is a great alternative to getting all of the diseases of aging that come with inadequate hormones.

The menstrual flow is just a minor inconvenience when you compare it to what may happen if you don't choose to adequately replace your hormones in a rhythmic manner.

Treatments for cancer are certainly no picnic. I would rather have my period than increase my cancer risk.

Not being able to walk is a real drag. I would rather have my period than to become so osteoporotic that the bones in my spine collapse.

Not being able to think or remember anything is not my cup of tea. I would rather have my period than to get Alzheimer's.

Double by-pass surgery is not for me. I would rather have my period than to develop heart disease.

I celebrate with a, "Whoo-hoo!" from the bathroom on the first day of every period. Perverse? No! I am grateful for the freedom of disease provided me by this monthly cleansing. Which do you choose, ladies? Period or disease?

The Wiley Protocol® may help you to heal. If you have any of the breast cancer risk factors listed below, cyclic BHRT (the Wiley Protocol®) may help you to heal your body so that you don't get breast cancer.

You are more susceptible to breast cancer if you:

- **Never breastfed.**[64]
- **Were never pregnant.**
- **Were only pregnant late in your life.**
- **Used synthetic female hormones (birth control pills, Premarin).**[65]
- **Went into puberty early.**
- **Went into menopause late.**
- **Have had toxic exposure (chemicals like dioxin).**
- **Have a lot of xenoestrogens in your body (plastics, cosmetics).**[66]

15: How to Prevent Cancer

TREATMENT OF BREAST CANCER WILL NOT REMOVE THE CONDITIONS THAT CAUSED IT. Surgically removing the breast, X-ray radiation therapy, and chemotherapy will not remove the conditions that caused the breast cancer in the first place. The remaining breast or other organs may still become cancerous. Radiation and chemotherapy are traumatic treatments that injure the immune system and tissues, weakening you, and increasing risk for cancer and other diseases.

To remove the conditions that cause cancer, it is necessary to improve your ability to metabolize (break down and use) estrogen well, optimize hormones, and detoxify the body. You can do this by avoiding the intake of horse and synthetic estrogens, decreasing your intake of xenoestrogens (plastics, pesticides, etc.), detoxifying the liver, and cleansing the colon. Improving your diet, maintaining good body weight, and regular exercise could reduce cancer by 30% to 40% or more.[67]

Traditional medical doctors always insist that you get a mammogram. Mammograms traumatize the breast cells and expose you to ionizing radiation, both of which have been proven to be *causes* of breast cancer.[68] [69] [70] Newer, better, gentler scans for breast cancer include breast imaging and thermography. Self breast exams are the most important measure to screen for lumps. Ultrasounds of breast, ovaries, and uterus are also important.

Be aware of new daily symptoms (for 2-3 months) of ovarian cancer which include bloating, abdominal pain, getting full faster after eating, and having to urinate frequently.[71] See your doctor if you have these symptoms. Get pap smears regularly.

Get an Estrogen Metabolism Test! Traditional doctors won't know what you are talking about if you mention an estrogen metabolism test. But there *are* a few progressive doctors out there who know that good estrogen metabolism is critical in preventing cancer. It is important that both men and women be tested. The only safe way to replace deficient estrogen is to measure how it is being broken down and eliminated by getting an estrogen metabolism test and then to correct any problems. To do this, you send in a first morning urine test to a lab. Metametrix lab[72] does an "Estronex" profile that will tell how you are metabolizing your estrogen. Estrogen metabolism testing is not available through community or hospital laboratories. According to

Joe Swartz, MD, a family practitioner in Boulder, CO, the vast *majority* (greater than 90%) of estrogen metabolism tests that he sees are abnormal. He relates this to xenoestrogen toxicity. Males are at risk for prostate cancer when they have abnormal estrogen metabolism.

Reduce stress for good estrogen metabolism.

DIM (di-indol-methane) normalizes estrogen metabolism

with no side effects.[73] [74] Taking appropriate amounts of di-indole methane (DIM) is the most important treatment to improve estrogen metabolism.[75] [76] [77] You can get it in the health food store.

Prevent cancer by eating cruciferous vegetables such as bok choy, broccoli, Brussels sprouts, cabbage, cauliflower, kale, kohlrabi, mustard, rutabagas, and turnips.[78] These cruciferous vegetables will be broken down into DIM by stomach acid. If you don't have enough stomach acid, supplement with betaine hydrochloride. DIM has been tested in humans and found to be safe and efficacious in inducing death of cervical cancer cells.[79] Even when taken at dosages of ten times the recommended amounts for assisting in estrogen metabolism, DIM has been found to be safe, with no side effects.

Improve your digestion. Health begins in the gut. Get

tested for parasites and other infectious diseases at specialty labs. If you have gall bladder problems, do the liver/gall bladder flush (internet) and use protective healing herbs. An overgrowth of yeast and bacteria in the gut may be treated by using probiotics (like lactobacillus), which can be found in the refrigerator at the health food store. Improve the digestion with betaine HCl and/or digestive enzymes if they are deficient, and reduce the intake of sugar, high carbohydrate meals, and refined or processed food.

Eat foods high in glucaric acid. Calcium D-Glucarate

(health food store) can greatly improve estrogen metabolism. Calcium D-Glucarate in certain foods inhibits cancer development.[80] These foods include apples, Brussels sprouts, cabbage, bean sprouts, broccoli, oranges, and lettuce. It is easily taken as a supplement.

Good oils improve estrogen metabolism.[81] Fish

and flax oil are also a good way to reduce inflammation.[82]

Improve mitochondrial function. People who have

chronic fatigue and fibromyalgia usually have mitochondrial dysfunction or loss of mitochondria (powerhouses of the cells). Mitochondrial mutations are found in many cancers. You can improve mitochondrial function with B vitamins, amino acids, alpha-lipoic acid, acetyl-L-carnitine, quercetin, resveratrol, and Co Q-10 (health food store).[83] You may be able to regenerate mitochondria with Xymogen's[84] "Mitochondrial Renewal Kit."

16: Testosterone, for Men *and* Women

TESTOSTERONE IS THE MAJOR MALE SEX HORMONE. Men have 10 to 40 times more than women.

Men are reluctant to discuss declining libido with their doctors without their wife's urging. Testosterone raises libido and is an antidepressant for both men and women. It is necessary to build strong bones. It increases the ratio of lean muscle mass to body fat. It increases sexual thoughts and fantasies. Testosterone increases the desire to be alone, assertiveness, aggression, and self-confidence. It drops when losing, being a vegetarian, eating a low-fat diet, and with stress. It increases when winning, thinking about sex or having sex, eating meat, and exercising. Testosterone is higher in the morning and lower at night, vacillating in between.

When testosterone is very high, men become irritable and want to be left alone. High levels may be associated with psychotic behavior and violent crime. Levels fluctuate in 15-20 minute cycles. An irritable man's mood may improve fifteen or twenty minutes later when testosterone levels drop. Animals whose testosterone is high will mark and aggressively defend their territory.

Testosterone decreases with age in both men and women. Levels begin dropping after age 30 and drop off drastically in men after age 60. 30% of U.S. men aged 60-70 have low testosterone. 70% of U.S. men aged 70-80 have low testosterone. There is very little testosterone in U.S. males after age 80. There are between 4-5 million American males with low testosterone. Only 5-10% of them receive testosterone therapy.

Both men and women may benefit from supplemental testosterone when levels are low. Testosterone is used to treat low sex drive and is FDA-approved for HRT in combination with estrogen for menopausal women and for andropausal men. Testosterone replacement improves mood, thinking, muscle mass, belly fat, thinning skin, and frailty (all signs of aging). Optimizing testosterone levels leads to lowered cholesterol, increased libido, and decreased risk of developing diabetes.[85] Compounding pharmacies can make a cream using testosterone with or without DHEA that is rubbed into the skin once a day.

Studies are conflicting as to the risk of testosterone use in females and breast cancer.[86][87][88][89] Caution must be advised until we are sure of its safety.

Adrenal exhaustion may lead to low testosterone in women. Women *who have low levels of testosterone* may benefit from testosterone replacement. It increases muscle mass, strength, and increases bone mineral density.[90]

Adding testosterone may be helpful, but may make problems worse if estrogen dominance is present. Testosterone is converted into estrogen by fat, especially belly fat. Therefore, supplementation of testosterone can raise estrogen levels. This will diminish the effects of the testosterone.

Doctors may confuse estrogen dominance with low testosterone. It is important to measure estrogen and testosterone levels when supplementing with testosterone.

Don't take too much testosterone or you'll feel great for a month and then crash. When taking amounts of testosterone that are too high, the cells will become resistant to taking in any more testosterone and then refuse to take it in at all. Taking breaks from the testosterone allows the cells to better absorb the testosterone when you do take it again.

Maca is an herb used to boost testosterone levels. The effects of this Peruvian "ginseng" may be quite dramatic.

Excess DHT. DHT is a form of testosterone that causes male secondary sex characteristics like deep voice, facial hair, and hair loss. High DHT levels are associated with enlarging the prostate gland and may lead to benign prostatic hyperplasia (BPH) and prostate cancer.

Some DHT is good because it gets rid of unwanted and cancerous cells, much like progesterone does in women. But in excess, this hormone may cause thinning hair, acne, facial hair, and lowered voice. Excess DHT damages healthy hair follicles, causing baldness in both men and women. Baldness affects men more than women because men have more testosterone that may be changed into DHT.

Testosterone is made into DHT. So be careful not to take too much testosterone, as you don't want to make too much DHT.

Protect against prostate disease and excess DHT by using these herbs: stinging nettle, saw palmetto, Pygeum africanum, and green tea extract. Pumpkin seeds are excellent. Other helpful supplements include: pycnogenol, omega-3 fatty acids, L-lysine, selenium, Vitamin E, minerals (*zinc*), antioxidants, grape seed extract, and gamma Linolenic Acid (GLA)

17: How to Deal with Andropause

ANDROPAUSE OCCURS WHEN A MAN'S TESTOSTERONE DROPS. Men don't like to think about losing their virility, and usually will seek treatment only at their wife's urging. Andropause approaches more slowly than female menopause, but the long-term consequences are just as deadly. Testosterone decline begins at 30 and drops severely with age.

Symptoms of untreated andropause include:
- **Men don't have as much energy.**
- **They can't think as well.**
- **Muscles are weaker.**
- **Joints ache.**
- **They are depressed and moody.**
- **They lose sexual desire and function.**
- **They often get fat,** especially around the middle. Enzymes in this fat turn their testosterone into estrogen.
- **Decreased testosterone.** Half of healthy men between the ages of 50-70 will have testosterone levels below the lowest level seen in healthy men who are 20-40.[91] A healthy 60-year-old would be a sick 25-year-old. To add to the problem, average (regardless of age) testosterone levels are declining world-wide. Perhaps it is being caused by environmental pollution and xenoestrogens.[92]
- **Death.**[93] In andropause, there is increased aging of the heart and brain. There are more heart attacks and strokes. Ironically, men resist getting testosterone replacement therapy for fear of getting cancer. But, in reality, testosterone *protects* them against cancer.[94] Optimal testosterone levels are *not* associated with an increase in prostate cancer.[95] [96]
- **Decreased Growth Hormone.** Drop in GH causes decreased bone mass and density, decreased muscle mass, and increased fat by up to 40%. It also causes shrinkage in kidneys, stomach, small intestine, liver, and spleen with decreased immune resilience.[97]
- **Decreased DHEA production** accentuates the effects of testosterone deficiency. Its loss increases weight, depression, and decreases sex drive.

- **Memory and intelligence decrease.** Dementia and Alzheimer's increase.
- **Performance anxiety** occurs when the male becomes anxious about his performance in sex. Adding to the loss of testosterone, he may also have narrowed penile arteries caused by atherosclerosis and erectile dysfunction from blood pressure or heart medications, alcohol and/or cigarettes. These constrict blood flow to his penis. His menopausal wife may be demanding, irritable, and disinterested in sex. Fears of being able to perform sexually may become self-fulfilling prophecy, causing avoidance of sex and loss of self-esteem, both of which result in low testosterone.
- **Behavior directed toward raising testosterone levels.** Andropause is accompanied by problems like performance anxiety, marital discord, job dissatisfaction, and self-perceived loss of importance, especially if his wife makes more money. Testosterone levels drop even further when he feels worthless. He may try to raise testosterone levels by enhancing his status. His car is a symbol of his success in the world. He might buy an expensive SUV, a red sports car convertible, or a Harley. Dying the grey hair away might help him look younger. Scalp implants or a toupee may give the illusion of youth. An affair with a younger woman would prove that he hasn't lost his virility. He may pick fights with his family and co-workers. He may move to another place hoping that testosterone will return to normal levels when he is alone. All of his behavior is a short-lived attempt to raise testosterone levels. Nothing he can do will work in the long run, except for BHRT.
- **Self-destructive behavior.** Testosterone-deficient males feel that they have lost the battle of life to younger, more powerful males. The worst-case scenario ends in suicide. These males search for any small victories to help bring up their testosterone. If they aren't successful, they become self-destructive, perhaps taking up smoking if they don't smoke already, drinking more alcohol, or taking drugs to ease the pain.
- **Other sexual problems.** Erection takes longer. Erections do not occur with fantasies or sight, but require mechanical stimulation. There aren't as many morning erections. Erections are not as firm. The need to have orgasm diminishes or disappears. There is longer recovery time between orgasms. The force of ejaculation is less. The desire for and frequency of

masturbation decreases. The testicles shrink and don't bunch up as much when sexually aroused.

- **Visible changes** appear as wrinkles, loss of muscle mass, and loss of height due to loss of bone density and weakened connective tissue.
- **Grumpy old man.** Mood deteriorates.
- **Shift in estrogen/testosterone ratio.** As testosterone drops, much of what is left is changed into estrogen. This shift towards more estrogen and less testosterone may cause him to become less dominant and more receptive in his relationship.
- **Erectile Dysfunction (E.D.)** is the inability to obtain and maintain an erection sufficient for sexual intercourse. It affects 75% of all American men who are older than 75. Erectile dysfunction is often associated with poor cardiovascular health. Viagra and related drugs and oxytocin are effective treatments for E.D.

If you are experiencing any of these changes, see your doctor.

He may be able to help you. He will help you to evaluate lifestyle and meds, treat depression, and then to consider whether to begin testosterone replacement therapy (TRT). Causes of low male hormones can be determined and discussed with your doctor.

The first thing to do is to address your lifestyle.

If you smoke and/or drink and/or are overweight, realize that you are jeopardizing your life. Exercise, see an anti-aging physician, and eat live foods.

Cardiovascular disease is the biggest cause of sexual dysfunction.

Find out if the meds you are taking are affecting your sexual performance and start a cardiac rehab program.

Depression may be disguised as chronic anger, irritability, and hostility.

Job loss, demotion, and approach of retirement may be depressing. Seek therapy if necessary. If you must take antidepressants, do so after BHRT is optimal, and find out if the antidepressants will affect sexual performance. Seek natural alternatives first. Educate and treat yourself if necessary.

Take the right amount of testosterone.

When testosterone is given to men who have abdominal fat, their abdominal fat may increase, because enzymes in the fat turn the testosterone into estrogen. Then anastrozole (Arimidex) is sometimes given to stop the estrogen formation. Calcium D-Glucarate is very helpful.

Enlarged breasts and belly fat are caused by too much estrogen. As men become more estrogen-dominant (in relation to testosterone), through taking in xenoestrogens, production of estrogen from body fat, and with the loss of testosterone caused by aging, they will develop breast enlargement. Estrogen dominance may also cause prostate inflammation and swelling. Lifestyle changes may be enough to correct the problem.[98] If testosterone levels are still low after improving lifestyle, begin testosterone replacement therapy. Get an estrogen metabolism test. Improve any bad estrogen metabolism.[99]

Testosterone replacement for men is safe and extremely beneficial.

- Testosterone decreases inflammation and cholesterol.[100]
- Testosterone improves cardiac function.[101] [102] [103]
- It improves symptoms of coronary artery disease.[104] [105]
- It normalizes blood pressure.[106]
- It improves glucose and decreases belly fat.[107]
- Testosterone improves mood even when drugs don't.[108]
- It improves body composition--more muscle, less fat.[109]
- It reverses osteoporosis.
- It may improve osteo- and rheumatoid arthritis.
- It does not cause prostate cancer.[110] [111] [112] [113]
- It doesn't hurt the prostate.[114] (Increased estrogen may produce prostatic symptoms.)
- It improves blood flow in the brain.[115]
- It may prevent Alzheimer's disease.[116]
- It restores sex drive, orgasm, nocturnal erections, and libido.[117]
- Alzheimer's patients improve with testosterone.[118]
- It improves cognitive function.[119] [120]
- It increases GH secretion by 10-20%.[121]
- It improves and may resolve erectile dysfunction.[122] [123]
- It improves stamina, cardiac pump function, and sexual function.

Prostate: Every man who lives long enough will develop benign or malignant prostatic cancer (usually microscopic). There is a 92% incidence at 92 years. Activators of microscopic cancer are poor estrogen metabolism, increased insulin levels, and all immune impairments.

Supplements that prevent prostate disease include:

- Vitamin E.[124]
- Selenium.
- Soy diets.
- Saw palmetto.
- Pygeum africanum.
- Pumpkin seed.
- Nettle.
- Omega-3's.
- Antioxidants.
- Minerals (zinc).
- Beta-sitosterol.
- DIM.
- Sabal (homeopathic).

To improve erectile dysfunction (E.D.):

Supplements should be used regularly and you should discontinue drugs that increase E.D. (beta-blockers), drugs that increase prolactin, SSRI's, and chronic antihistamine use. Healthy sex is important in the prevention of erectile dysfunction.

- Oxytocin. [125]
- L-arginine.
- Gingko.
- Tribulus.
- Maca.
- Ginseng.
- Muira puama.
- Niacin.
- Viagra (Last resort, as this is a toxic drug).

Let's look next at what else we need to do to balance our hormones.

18: Cleanse Toxins, Balance Hormones

Xenoestrogens are environmental poisons that act like estrogen.

They are a major reason for the epidemic of hormonal problems. We must constantly be on guard to keep them out of our bodies and cleanse them from our bodies. They disrupt the actions of estrogens formed in our bodies.[126] These toxins include pesticides, synthetic hormones fed to animals, petrochemicals, solvents, plastics, and cosmetics. They are major factors in the increase in breast cancer,[127] and they lower sperm count.[128] They are much more potent than the estrogen the body makes, contributing to estrogen excess in both men and women. The body can't easily get rid of them. They may damage DNA and lead to breast, ovarian,[129] testicular and prostate cancer.[130] [131] They cause genetic mutations that are passed on from generation to generation.[132] Men become feminized. Drinking water from plastic bottles is a major source.[133] Five billion pounds of pesticide, herbicide, and other biocides are added each year to our planet's soil, water, and air. No one can avoid being intoxicated with them.

Toxicity will prevent every other strategy from working. Toxins put the brakes on your ability to heal and lose weight.[134]

First, stop putting external toxins into your body in any way you can. If you don't put them in, you don't have to work to get them out. Quit using toxic stimulants such as caffeine, tobacco, sodas, diet pills, and alcohol. Also give up all unnecessary pharmaceuticals and synthetic hormones. Stop eating all canned, refined, and processed food. Read the labels and avoid buying anything with nitrites,[135] hydrogenated oils,[136] trans fats,[137] and preservatives. When buying meat, fish, and fowl, get it as fresh as possible. If it does not say that it was raised without antibiotics and/or hormones, don't buy it if you can find alternatives without antibiotics or hormones. Caged poultry and farm-raised fish should be strictly avoided because they are raised in extremely toxic environments,[138] given drugs, and fed unnatural food.[139] [140] Fluoride is in our drinking water and some toothpaste. It's a poison.[141] Filter your water and use natural toothpaste without fluoride. Avoid chlorinated and brominated pools. You can detoxify with iodine, Celtic sea salt, and pink salt from the Himalayas. Drink lots of purified water.

An often-overlooked toxicity is electromagnetic radiation (EMR). EMR may cause sleeplessness, weight gain and general fatigue. It is also associated with cancer.[142] If at all possible, don't live near high voltage power lines on big steel towers. These huge power lines are very disruptive to health. Connect any electrical devices in your bedroom to power strips and turn them off before you go to sleep. Don't sleep with your head near any outlets. Keep your cell phone far from your bed.

Second, cleanse the large intestine. The body uses the large intestine as the primary organ of cleansing and detoxification. Skin is second and lung is third. Help it along by eating lots of natural fiber, by taking supplemental fiber (psyllium, pectin, and/or other natural fibers), and bentonite. Be careful. If diseases are too advanced, fiber may be very irritating. Fiber is a structural component of many plants. Increasing fiber intake has many health benefits.[143] [144] Fiber helps to remove excess estrogen from the bodies of both men and women reducing cancer risk.[145]

Colonics and enemas are a great way to detoxify,[146] even removing heavy metals. Colonics and enemas decrease the time that stool remains in the colon. This gives your body less time to absorb toxic compounds that are sitting there.

Third, detox through the skin. Use a sauna to sweat out the toxins stored in fat.[147] [148] A portable, collapsible far infrared (FIR) is a comfortable way to detox, as your head sticks out through the top. With your head remaining cool, you can tolerate the heat on the rest of your body enough to really get a good sweat going. With openings for your arms, you can read or type while sitting in the sauna for several hours each day.

Fourth, cleanse and support the liver. Coffee enemas became established into medicine when Dr. Max Gerson began using them to treat cancer patients in the 1930's.[149] Lam et al offered scientific support by showing that substances in coffee detoxify carcinogens by neutralizing free radicals, which have been implicated in initiating cancer.[150] Taking organic chlorella a half hour before the coffee enema will help bind toxic substances in the bile so that they can be eliminated.[151] [152] [153]

Remove mercury and other heavy metals. For many people, their highest toxic burden is mercury poisoning. Stop eating mercury-containing foods such as tuna and other large fish. Remove mercury fillings (amalgams). Other common heavy metal toxicity includes arsenic and aluminum, which has been implicated in Alzheimer's disease.[154] If you have heavy metal poisoning, identified by chelated urine tests for heavy metals, you may need to undergo chelation treatments until levels are reduced sufficiently.

19: Lower Stress to Balance Hormones

Stress[155] PLAYS HAVOC WITH HORMONAL BALANCE IN BOTH WOMEN AND MEN.

It is important to minimize stress.

Mental stress includes financial pressures, information overloading, time urgency, and the pressure to multi-task.

Emotional stress comes from the breakdown of the family unit, relationship difficulties, performance pressure, boring jobs, and traumatic events that result in post-traumatic stress disorder.

Physical stress may come from over-exercising, but more often comes from under-exercising. Faulty diet and toxicity add to the physical stress.

Many people have adrenal exhaustion.[156] The adrenals are small organs that sit on top of the kidneys. The adrenals' primary job is to deal with stress. People whose adrenals are exhausted often work 60-80 hours a week. *They are tired but won't take the time to rest.* They keep working hard until the continued stress burns out their organs.

Many people are tired and in overwhelm. This is feeling "tired and wired." They can't rest because they have to pay the mortgage. These people often arrive at the doctor's office with nervousness, hormonal problems, low libido, and low muscle tone and strength. They may have memory loss, poor immune function, low energy, and bad mood. They often have fatigue, anxiety, and food cravings.

When the stress is prolonged, it may lead to adrenal fatigue and eventually to adrenal exhaustion, neither of which are recognized by traditional doctors as treatable medical conditions. As the adrenals become burned out, they can't support the normal activities of life.

Stress may make you fat.[157] Sustained stress causes the body to refuel when it doesn't need to refuel. Stress breaks down the body. This results in burning up the building blocks of the body and creating abdominal fat by stimulating the appetite.[158]

Stress may make you sick and kill you.[159] Stress is responsible for weight gain (especially belly fat), blood sugar Imbalance, thinning skin, muscle wasting, and aging.

DHEA will be stolen from its job in making sex hormones to deal with the stress in both women and men. When you are under chronic stress, you are breaking down more than building up. You are accelerating the aging process.

If DHEA is low, supplement with it. When we don't have enough DHEA, we get sick more easily and cannot deal with stress as well. It is important to keep levels up because the sex hormones are formed from it. DHEA improves quality of life and longevity. When DHEA is optimized, it promotes a sense of well-being. As it is depleted, carbohydrate cravings increase, leading to more weight gain.

Take sulfur to store the DHEA. MSM will do the trick. If people are deficient in DHEA, leg hair stops growing. Leg hair may be completely absent or stop north of the ankles, as if the socks were rubbing the hair off. If leg hair is absent, test DHEA and adrenal function. DHEA can be taken orally in supplements, but the most effective way to take it is by rubbing on a cream prescribed by your doctor. This cream may also contain testosterone if you are low.

- **DHEA increases sex drive,** more in women than it does in men. DHEA decreases cholesterol and promotes bone growth.
- **DHEA causes weight loss** by making you warmer, causing you to burn more energy. It targets fat loss around the abdomen.
- **DHEA builds collagen.** By having sufficient reserves of DHEA you decrease wrinkles and the need for orthopedic surgery when you get older. To test your collagen, pinch the back of your hand to see how fast your skin springs back. If it is slow, test DHEA and rebuild collagen.[160]
- **DHEA keeps people sexually attractive,** improves quality of life, and reduces mortality from all causes. It protects against breast and other cancers. It improves cognition and protects the immune system. DHEA builds tissue. It stimulates the immune system, and maintains tissue elasticity and repair.
- **DHEA improves memory.** DHEA also acts as an antidepressant.
- **DHEA lowers heart disease and protects** against midlife changes. It is used in the treatment of aging, menopause, andropause, immune deficiencies, breast cancer, AIDS, and osteoporosis.

Pregnenolone also may be stolen to deal with stress in both women and men. Pregnenolone is formed from cholesterol. Pregnenolone is used to form DHEA, progesterone, and other sex hormones. Stress steals the pregnenolone and results in obesity, hypothyroidism, inflammation, hypertension, and gall bladder problems.

Supplement with pregnenolone if you are low. Pregnenolone is a potent memory enhancer. It improves mental fatigue and helps with focus and concentration. It affects mood. It is inhibited by trans fats. Weight gain may occur when it is low.

Eat plenty of cholesterol to make adequate sex hormones. Don't believe the media hype. Cholesterol-lowering drugs cause multiple health problems. You need to eat plenty of cholesterol-containing foods to insure adequate pregnenolone production. These foods include butter, shellfish, eggs, and meat.

Don't deprive yourself of these important cholesterol-containing foods. Eat cholesterol so that you can make the hormones that you need to be healthy. Do all things in moderation.

You can reframe stress and heal. It is all in your attitude. By recognizing that you have done many things successfully, and that you can build on those successes, you can realize that you can deal with any new stress successfully.

Humans rehearse and replay traumatic events. This replaying causes all the same reactions as if it is actually happening again. We re-live it in our mind and body. The next time you find yourself replaying a trauma, complete the story, but this time, picture yourself as coming out victorious. Beat up your pillow, yell, scream, fight, get away, or do whatever it takes to finish the incomplete flight or fight reaction. Don't leave yourself stuck where you are now, which is the one place you don't want to be, unable to fight or flee, stuck in the other "f," "frozen" in a time long past. Release frozen trauma reactions if you want to move on with your life.

Therapists who help people to overcome stress disorders include those who use Peter Levine's "Somatic Experiencing" (SE),[161] John Upledger's "Somato-Emotional Release" (SER),[162] "Eye Movement Desensitization and Reprocessing" (EMDR),[163] and shamanic soul retrieval as taught by Gwilda Wiyaka at her "Path Home" shamanic practitioner training.[164]

Re-prioritize your life as much as you possibly can so that you are not under so much stress. This is one of the most important things that you can do to balance your hormones.

20: What about the Money, Honey?

BEFORE I STARTED BHRT, I HAD SOME LARGE HEALTH CARE BILLS TO PAY, AND I DIDN'T HAVE INSURANCE.

My heart malfunction cost $2000. They gave me beta-blockers which I hated and threw into the trash. I just had to take it easy until I got better. The cardiologist never mentioned the hormone deficit that was responsible for the heart problem.

The surgery for the skin cancer cost me $4000. The dermatologist never mentioned the hormone deficit that allowed the cancer to develop.

The cataract surgery cost me $7000. The eye surgeon never mentioned the hormone deficit that allowed this cataract to develop.

The thyroid problem cost about $600 a year. Nobody ever mentioned the adrenal and sex hormone deficit that allowed my thyroid to fail.

The adrenal exhaustion cost me my livelihood and my joy in being active. Nobody ever mentioned the hormone deficit or bad lifestyle (over-exercising and under-eating) that allowed the adrenal exhaustion to develop.

BHRT costs me $85 a month and about $300 a year in doctors bills. I consider these bioidentical hormones, good lifestyle, and the vitamins and supplements that I take (about $2000 a year) to BE my insurance. I am insuring myself against all of the illnesses that would happen if I weren't taking hormones and supplements.

To pay for insurance, just for myself, it would cost about $10,000 a year. And it wouldn't pay for much anyway. You have to argue with these insurance people over and over to get any bills paid, and they always have some excuse why they won't pay.

If you have some chronic disease, you may need insurance to cover your costs. But realize that bioidentical hormones may help you to heal from your chronic disease.

You can try to persuade your insurance to pay for BHRT. After all, they do pay for artificial hormones like birth control pills, Premarin, Prempro, and Viagra. But even if your insurance won't pay for BHRT, you should realize that the small cost to you is well worth the future health gains and avoidance of disease that you will reap.

21: How to Choose the Right Physician.

MOST DOCTORS TREAT MENOPAUSE **WITH DRUGS.** Traditional doctors treat menopausal symptoms with antidepressants for the depression, thyroid meds if the blood tests show hypothyroidism, and Premarin plus or minus Provera for hormone replacement therapy for a limited amount of time.

Even though Premarin and Provera have been proven to be dangerous, [165] [166] [167] [168] they are standard of care because that is what peer doctors are prescribing and what has been used for years. Traditional doctors (most primary-care physicians, endocrinologists, internists, etc.) will diagnose and treat only *extreme* hormonal imbalances.

The standard of care is gradually shifting to bioidentical hormones, based on the number of physicians who recognize the dangers of drugs like Premarin and Provera and the safety and efficacy of bioidentical hormones. State-of-the-art physicians are now prescribing bioidentical hormones. Anti-aging physicians and alternative medical physicians treat mild, moderate, and severe hormonal dysfunctions *preventing* the deterioration to extreme hormonal imbalances.

If you are unable to find a doctor in your area who is willing to treat you with bioidentical hormones for your hormonal deficiencies and imbalances, be they mild, moderate, or severe, find a doctor associated with the American Academy of Anti-Aging Medicine (A4M)[169] or American College for Advancement in Medicine (ACAM).[170] These anti-aging and functional medicine doctors are practicing state-of-the-art medicine, the medicine conservative physicians will be practicing in forty years. These doctors will be able to order the tests that you need. If you are looking for a doctor who will prescribe the Wiley Protocol®, you can find one on the internet at www.thewileyprotocol.com.

When you look for a doctor, look for a caring person with a warm heart. Avoid doctors whose only concern is to maximize profits for their HMO. Sidestep also the greedy ones, who maximize profits for themselves. Beware of any who feel that they are superior to you, "the patient," or those who are simply lazy or incompetent. Your goal is to find a physician whose motivation comes from the heart, works hard to be of service to you, who will approach you as a unique person, and will travel *with* you on your quest for health.

22: What You Need to Do Now

YOU NEED TO GET TO BED EARLY. It won't do you as much good to replace your hormones unless you improve your lifestyle as well. Go to bed by 9:00. Taking time-released melatonin[171] before bed is a great idea. Keep your bedroom totally dark. Your brain makes melatonin in the dark. The hours from 9 pm to midnight are critically important for you to be sleeping if you want to get your hormones balanced. If you don't have this sleep-wake cycle timed to go to sleep at sunset, your hormones will be unbalanced.[172]

Keep your carbohydrate intake low. Eating too many carbs and foods that quickly raise your blood sugar[173] (sugar, white flour, and white foods in general) leads to insulin resistance. Then your cells won't be able to use the estrogen you are taking. Eat only small portions of carbohydrates buffered with plenty of protein and good fats.[174] Totally remove sugar and processed foods from your diet.

Have no fear. We have seen that hormones made by pharmaceutical companies are bad. They harm the body. They are poor substitutes for the real, bioidentical hormones made by compounding pharmacies.

We have also learned that BHRT for women is best used transdermally in a rhythmic dosing schedule that mimics the monthly hormonal amounts and surges of young, healthy women. This is the way to avoid the ravages of old age. When men's testosterone levels drop with age, testosterone replacement is safe and beneficial, protecting them from the diseases common to aging men.

Instead of fearing the use of bioidentical hormones, it would be wiser to fear the consequences that result from the lack of hormones as we age. BHRT can help us to age without infirmity. I am personally very grateful for this gift of BHRT and hope that this book finds its way into the hands of those who are able to accept and use this information.

Read my "Secrets" book to learn more. For more detailed information, please read my last book. There you will find treatment plans that can be used by you and your doctor to balance all of your hormones. It is an excellent reference. Please pick up a copy of <u>Secrets about Bioidentical Hormones to Lose Fat and Prevent Cancer, Heart Disease, Menopause, and Andropause, by Optimizing Adrenals, Thyroid, Estrogen, Progesterone, Testosterone, and Growth Hormone!</u>

References

[1] Moskowitz D. A comprehensive review of the safety and efficacy of bioidentical hormones for the management of menopause and related health risks. *Altern Med Rev. 2006 Sep;11(3):208-23.*

[2] Wood CE, Register TC, Lees CJ, Chen H, Kimrey S, Cline JM. Effects of estradiol with micronized progesterone or medroxyprogesterone acetate on risk markers for breast cancer in postmenopausal monkeys. *Breast Cancer Res Treat. 2007 Jan;101(2):125-34.*

[3] Hargrove JT, Maxson WS, Wentz AC, Burnett LS. Menopausal hormone replacement therapy with continuous daily oral micronized estradiol and progesterone. *Obstet Gynecol. 1989 Apr;73(4):606-12.*

[4] Stampfer MJ, Colditz GA, Willett WC, Manson JE, Rosner B, Speizer FE, Hennekens CH. Postmenopausal estrogen therapy and cardiovascular disease. Ten-year follow-up from the nurses' health study. *N Engl J Med. 1991 Sep 12;325(11):756-62.*

[5] Grady D, Rubin SM, Petitti DB, Fox CS, Black D, Ettinger B, Ernster VL, Cummings SR. Hormone therapy to prevent disease and prolong life in postmenopausal women. *Ann Intern Med. 1992 Dec 15;117(12):1016-37.*

[6] Brinton LA, Hoover RN. Estrogen replacement therapy and endometrial cancer rrisk: unresolved issues. The Endometrial Cancer Collaborative Group. *Obstet Gynecol. 1993 Feb;81(2):265-71.*

[7] Grady D, Gebretsadik T, Kerlikowske K, Ernster V, Petitti D. Hormone replacement therapy and endometrial cancer risk: a meta-analysis. *Obstet Gynecol.1995 Feb;85(2):304-13.*

[8] Comerci JT Jr, Fields AL, Runowicz CD, Goldberg GL. Continuous low-dose combined hormone replacement therapy and the risk of endometrial cancer. *Gynecol Oncol. 1997 Mar;64(3):425-30.*

[9] Cushing KL, Weiss NS, Voigt LF, McKnight B, Beresford SA. Risk of endometrial cancer in relation to use of low-dose, unopposed estrogens. *Obstet Gynecol. 1998 Jan;91(1):35-9.*

[10] Persson I, Yuen J, Bergkvist L, Schairer C. Cancer incidence and mortality in women receiving estrogen and estrogen-progestin replacement therapy--long-term follow-up of a Swedish cohort. *Int J Cancer. 1996 Jul 29;67(3):327-32.*

[11] Milliez J. [Non-surgical prevention of uterine cancer]. *Bull Acad Natl Med.1997 Oct;181(7):1415-31.*

[12] Elit L. Endometrial cancer. Prevention, detection, management, and follow up. *Can Fam Physician. 2000 Apr;46:887-92.*

[13] Physician's Desk Reference, 63rd edition. 2009. Physician's Desk Reference Inc. Montvale, N. J. p. 3217.

[14] Manson JE, Hsia J, Johnson KC, Rossouw JE, Assaf AR, Lasser NL, Trevisan M, Black HR, Heckbert SR, Detrano R, Strickland OL, Wong ND, Crouse JR, Stein E,Cushman M; Women's Health Initiative Investigators. Estrogen plus progestin and the risk of coronary heart disease. *N Engl J Med. 2003 Aug 7;349(6):523-34.*

[15] Hulley S, Grady D, Bush T, Furberg C, Herrington D, Riggs B, Vittinghoff E. Randomized trial of estrogen plus progestin for secondary prevention of coronary heart disease in postmenopausal women. Heart and Estrogen/progestin Replacement Study (HERS) Research Group. *JAMA. 1998 Aug 19;280(7):605-13.*

[16] Rossouw JE, Anderson GL, Prentice RL, LaCroix AZ, Kooperberg C, Stefanick ML, Jackson RD, Beresford SA, Howard BV, Johnson KC, Kotchen JM, Ockene J; Writing Group for the Women's Health Initiative Investigators. Risks and benefits of estrogen plus progestin in healthy postmenopausal women: principal results From the Women's Health Initiative randomized controlled trial. *JAMA. 2002 Jul 17;288(3):321-33.*

[17] Chlebowski RT, Anderson GL, Gass M, Lane DS, Aragaki AK, Kuller LH, Manson JE,

Stefanick ML, Ockene J, Sarto GE, Johnson KC, Wactawski-Wende J, Ravdin PM, Schenken R, Hendrix SL, Rajkovic A, Rohan TE, Yasmeen S, Prentice RL; WHI Investigators. Estrogen plus progestin and breast cancer incidence and mortality in postmenopausal women. *JAMA. 2010 Oct 20;304(15):1684-92.*

[18] Lee J, Hopkins V. *What Your Doctor May Not Tell You About Menopause.* New York, New York: Warner Books, 1996.

[19] Wiley TS, Taguchi J, Formby B. *Sex, Lies and Menopause.* New York, New York: Harper Collins Publishers, Inc. 2003.

[20] Moskowitz D. A comprehensive review of the safety and efficacy of bioidentical hormones for the management of menopause and related health risks. *Altern Med Rev. 2006 Sep;11(3):208-23.*

[21] Holtorf K. The bioidentical hormone debate: are bioidentical hormone (estradiol, estriol, and progesterone) safer or more efficacious than commonlyused synthetic versions in hormone replacement therapy? *Postgrad Med. 2009 Jan;121(1):73-85.*

[22] Ruiz AD, Daniels KR, Barner JC, Carson JJ, Frei CR. Effectiveness of Compounded Bioidentical Hormone Replacement Therapy: An Observational Cohort Study. *BMC Womens Health. 2011 Jun 8;11(1):27.*

[23] Formby B, Schmidt F. Efficacy of biorhythmic transdermal combined hormone treatment in relieving climacteric symptoms: a pilot study. *Int J Gen Med. 2011 Feb 28;4:159-63.*

[24] Wright YL. *Secrets about Bioidentical Hormones to Lose Fat and Prevent Cancer, Heart Disease, Menopause, and Andropause, by Optimizing Adrenals, Thyroid, Estrogen, Progesterone, Testosterone, and Growth Hormone!* Lulu.com. December 18, 2010. p. 56.

[25] Wright YL. *Secrets about Bioidentical Hormones to Lose Fat and Prevent Cancer, Heart Disease, Menopause, and Andropause, by Optimizing Adrenals, Thyroid, Estrogen, Progesterone, Testosterone, and Growth Hormone!* Lulu.com. December 18, 2010. p. 28.

[26] Wright YL. *Secrets about Bioidentical Hormones to Lose Fat and Prevent Cancer, Heart Disease, Menopause, and Andropause, by Optimizing Adrenals, Thyroid, Estrogen, Progesterone, Testosterone, and Growth Hormone!* Lulu.com. December 18, 2010. p. 48.

[27] Wright YL. *Secrets about Bioidentical Hormones to Lose Fat and Prevent Cancer, Heart Disease, Menopause, and Andropause, by Optimizing Adrenals, Thyroid, Estrogen, Progesterone, Testosterone, and Growth Hormone!* Lulu.com. December 18, 2010.

[28] Campagnoli C, Abbà C, Ambroggio S, Peris C. Pregnancy, progesterone and progestins in relation to breast cancer risk. *J Steroid Biochem Mol Biol. 2005 Dec;97(5):441-50.*

[29] Arevalo MA, Diz-Chaves Y, Santos-Galindo M, Bellini MJ, Garcia-Segura LM. SELECTIVE OESTROGEN RECEPTOR MODULATORS DECREASE THE INFLAMMATORY RESPONSE OF GLIAL CELLS. *J Neuroendocrinol. 2011 May 12.*

[30] Micevych P, Bondar G, Kuo J. Estrogen actions on neuroendocrine glia. *Neuroendocrinology. 2010;91(3):211-22.*

[31] Conaway E. Bioidentical hormones: an evidence-based review for primary careproviders. *J Am Osteopath Assoc. 2011 Mar;111(3):153-64.*

[32] Arrenbrecht S, Boermans AJ. Effects of transdermal estradiol delivered by a matrix patch on bone density in hysterectomized, postmenopausal women: a 2-year placebo-controlled trial. *Osteoporos Int. 2002;13(2):176-83.*

[33] Unsal A, Tozun M, Ayranci U. Prevalence of depression among postmenopausal women and related characteristics. *Climacteric. 2010 Oct 21.*

[34] Conaway E. Bioidentical hormones: an evidence-based review for primary careproviders. *J Am Osteopath Assoc. 2011 Mar;111(3):153-64.*

[35] Head KA. Estriol: safety and efficacy. *Altern Med Rev. 1998 Apr;3(2):101-13.*

[36] Lemon HM, Kumar PF, Peterson C, Rodriguez-Sierra JF, Abbo KM. Inhibition of radiogenic mammary carcinoma in rats by estriol or tamoxifen. *Cancer. 1989 May 1; 63(9):1685-92.*

[37] Weiderpass B. Low-potency oestrogen and risk of endometrial cancer: a case-control study. *Lancet 1999;353:1824-1828.*

[38] Monaco ME, Bolan G. Effects of estrone, estradiol, and estriol on hormone-responsive human breast cancer in long-term tissue culture. *Cancer Res. 1977 Jun;37(6):1901-7.*

[39] Van Haaften M, Donker GH, Sie-Go DM, Haspels AA, Thijssen JH. Biochemical and histological effects of vaginal estriol and estradiol applications on the endometrium, myometrium and vagina of postmenopausal women. *Gynecol Endocrinol. 1997 Jun;11(3):175-85.*

[40] Telang NT, Suto A, Wong GY, Osborne MP, Bradlow HL. Induction by estrogen metabolite 16 alpha-hydroxyestrone of genotoxic damage and aberrant proliferation in mouse mammary epithelial cells. *J Natl Cancer Inst. 1992 Apr 15;84(8):634-8.*

[41] Weiderpass B. Low-potency oestrogen and risk of endometrial cancer: a case-control study. *Lancet 1999;353:1824-1828.*

[42] Monaco ME, Bolan G. Effects of estrone, estradiol, and estriol on hormone-responsive human breast cancer in long-term tissue culture. *Cancer Res. 1977 Jun;37(6):1901-7.*

[43] Divi RL, Chang HC, Doerge DR. Anti-thyroid isoflavones from soybean: isolation, characterization, and mechanisms of action. *Biochem Pharmacol 1997 Nov 15 54:10 1087-96.*

[44] Ishizuki Y, Hirooka Y, Murata Y, Togashi K. The effects on the thyroid gland of soybeans administered experimentally in healthy subjects. *Nippon Naibunpi Gakkai Zasshi 1991 May 20 67:5 622-9 (Japanese).*

[45] Kumar A, Naidu PS, Seghal N, Padi SS. Neuroprotective effects of resveratrol against intracerebroventricular colchicine-induced cognitive impairment and oxidative stress in rats. *Pharmacology 2007;79:17-26.*

[46] Seely EW, Walsh BW, Gerhard MD, Williams GH. Estradiol with or without progesterone and ambulatory blood pressure in postmenopausal women. *Hypertension.1999 May;33(5):1190-4.*

[47] Salminen HS, Sääf ME, Johansson SE, Ringertz H, Strender LE. The effect of transvaginal estradiol on bone in aged women: a randomised controlled trial. *Maturitas. 2007 Aug 20;57(4):370-81.*

[48] Hargrove JT, Maxson WS, Wentz AC, Burnett LS. Menopausal hormone replacement therapy with continuous daily oral micronized estradiol and progesterone. *Obstet Gynecol. 1989 Apr;73(4):606-12.*

[49] Decensi A, Omodei U, Robertson C, Bonanni B, Guerrieri-Gonzaga A, Ramazzotto F, Johansson H, Mora S, Sandri MT, Cazzaniga M, Franchi M, Pecorelli S. Effect of transdermal estradiol and oral conjugated estrogen on C-reactive protein in retinoid-placebo trial in healthy women. *Circulation 2002 Sep 3:106(10):1224-8.*

[50] Wright YL. *Secrets about Bioidentical Hormones to Lose Fat and Prevent Cancer, Heart Disease, Menopause, and Andropause, by Optimizing Adrenals, Thyroid, Estrogen, Progesterone, Testosterone, and Growth Hormone!* Lulu.com. December 18, 2010. p. 27.

[51] Heerdt AS, Young CW, Borgen PI. Calcium glucarate as a chemopreventive agent in breast cancer. *Altern Med Rev. 2002 Aug; 7(4):336-9.*

[52] Heersche JN, Bellows CG, Ishida Y. The decrease in bone mass associated with aging and menopause. *J Prosthet Dent. 1998 Jan;79(1):14-6.*

[53] Voloshenyuk TG, Gardner JD. Estrogen improves TIMP-MMP balance and collagen distribution in volume-overloaded hearts of ovariectomized females. *Am J Physiol Regul Integr Comp Physiol. 2010 Aug;299(2):R683-93.*

[54] http://www.thewileyprotocol.com 805-565-7508

[55] Wiley TS, Formby B. *Lights Out.* New York, New York: Pocket Books, Simon & Schuster, Inc. 2000.

[56] Wiley TS, Taguchi J, Formby B. *Sex, Lies and Menopause.* New York, New York: Harper Collins Publishers, Inc. 2003.

[57] Micevych P, Bondar G, Kuo J. Estrogen actions on neuroendocrine glia. *Neuroendocrinology. 2010;91(3):211-22.*

[58] Micevych P, Kuo J, Christensen A. Physiology of membrane oestrogen receptor signalling

in reproduction. *J Neuroendocrinol. 2009 Mar;21(4):249-56.*

[59] Formby B, Wiley TS. Bcl-2, survivin and variant CD44 v7-v10 are downregulated and p53 is upregulated in breast cancer cells by progesterone: inhibition of cell growth and induction of apoptosis. *Mol Cell Biochem. 1999 Dec;202(1-2):53-61.*

[60] Formby B, Wiley TS. Progesterone inhibits growth and induces apoptosis in breast cancer cells: inverse effects on Bcl-2 and p53. *Ann Clin Lab Sci. 1998 Nov-Dec;28(6):360-9.*

[61] Horita K, Inase N, Miyake S, Formby B, Toyoda H, Yoshizawa Y. Progesterone induces apoptosis in malignant mesothelioma cells. *Anticancer Res. 2001 Nov-Dec;21(6A):3871-4.*

[62] Syed V, Ho SM. Progesterone-induced apoptosis in immortalized normal and malignant human ovarian surface epithelial cells involves enhanced expression of FasL. *Oncogene. 2003 Oct 9;22(44):6883-90.*

[63] Wright YL. *Secrets about Bioidentical Hormones to Lose Fat and Prevent Cancer, Heart Disease, Menopause, and Andropause, by Optimizing Adrenals, Thyroid, Estrogen, Progesterone, Testosterone, and Growth Hormone!* Lulu.com. December 18, 2010. p. 31.

[64] De Silva M, Senarath U, Gunatilake M, Lokuhetty D. Prolonged breastfeeding reduces risk of breast cancer in Sri Lankan women: a case-control study. *Cancer Epidemiol. 2010 Jun;34(3):267-73.*

[65] Okamoto Y, Liu X, Suzuki N, Okamoto K, Kim HJ, Laxmi YR, Sayama K, Shibutani S. Equine estrogen-induced mammary tumors in rats. *Toxicol Lett. 2010 Apr 1;193(3):224-8.*

[66] Torres-Mejía G, Angeles-Llerenas A. [Reproductive factors and breast cancer: principal findings in Latin America and the world]. *Salud Publica Mex. 2009;51 Suppl 2:s165-71. Spanish.*

[67] Amin AR, Kucuk O, Khuri FR, Shin DM. Perspectives for cancer prevention with natural compounds. *J Clin Oncol. 2009 Jun 1;27(16):2712-25.*

[68] Bailar JC 3rd. Mammography: a contrary view. *Ann Intern Med. 1976 Jan;84(1):77-84.*

[69] Thornton H. Breast screening seems driven by belief rather than evidence. *BMJ. 2002 Ma16;324(7338):677.*

[70] O'Connor MK, Li H, Rhodes DJ, Hruska CB, Clancy CB, Vetter RJ. Comparison of radiation exposure and associated radiation-induced cancer risks from mammography and molecular imaging of the breast. Med Phys. 2010 Dec;37(12):6187-98.

[71] Kim MK, Kim K, Kim SM, Kim JW, Park NH, Song YS, Kang SB. A hospital-based case-control study of identifying ovarian cancer using symptom index. *J Gynecol Oncol. 2009 Dec;20(4):238-42.*

[72] http://www.metametrix.com/   800-221-4640

[73] Jin Y, Zou X, Feng X. 3,3'-Diindolylmethane negatively regulates Cdc25A and induces a G2/M arrest by modulation of microRNA 21 in human breast cancer cells. *Anticancer Drugs. 2010 Oct;21(9):814-22.*

[74] Sepkovic DW, Stein J, Carlisle AD, Ksieski HB, Auborn K, Bradlow HL. Diindolylmethane inhibits cervical dysplasia, alters estrogen metabolism, and enhances immune response in the K14-HPV16 transgenic mouse model. *Cancer Epidemiol Biomarkers Prev. 2009 Nov;18(11):2957-64.*

[75] Chen I, McDougal A, Wang F, Safe S. Aryl hydrocarbon receptor-mediated antiiestrogenic and antitumorigenic activity of diindolylmethane. *Carcinogenesis 1998 Sep;19(9):1631-9.*

[76] Chang X, Tou JC, Hong C, Kim HA, Riby JE, Firestone GL, Bjeldanes LF. 3,3'-Diindolylmethane inhibits angiogenesis and the growth of transplantable human breast carcinoma in athymic mice. *Carcinogenesis. 2005 Apr;26(4):771-8.*

[77] Vivar OI, Saunier EF, Leitman DC, Firestone GL, Bjeldanes LF. Selective activation of estrogen receptor-beta target genes by 3,3'-diindolylmethane. *Endocrinology. 2010 Apr;151(4):1662-7. Epub 2010 Feb 16.*

[78] Fowke JH, Longcope C, Hebert JR. Brassica vegetable consumption shifts estrogen metabolism in healthy postmenopausal women. *Cancer Epidemiol Biomarkers Prev*

2000;9(8):773-9.

[79] Leong H, Firestone GL, Bjeldanes LF. Cytostatic effects of 3,3-diindolylmethane in human endometrial cancer cells result from an estrogen receptor-mediated increase in transforming growth factor-alpha expression. *Carcinogenesis. 2001 Nov;22(11):1809-17.*

[80] Hanausek M, Walaszek Z, Slaga TJ. Detoxifying cancer causing agents to prevent cancer. *Integr Cancer Ther. 2003 Jun;2(2):139-44.*

[81] Spector AA, Burns CP. Biological and therapeutic potential of membrane lipid modification in tumors. *Cancer Res. 1987 Sep 1;47(17):4529-37.*

[82] Lee JC, Krochak R, Blouin A, Kanterakis S, Chatterjee S, Arguiri E, Vachani A, Solomides CC, Cengel KA, Christofidou-Solomidou M. Dietary flaxseed prevents radiation-induced oxidative lung damage, inflammation and fibrosis in a mouse model of thoracic radiation injury. *Cancer Biol Ther. 2009 Jan;8(1):47-53.*

[83] Pollard PJ, Wortham NC, Tomlinson IP. The TCA cycle and tumorigenesis: the examples of fumarate hydratase and succinate dehydrogenase. *Ann Med. 2003;35(8):632-9.*

[84] http://www.xymogen.com/2008/index.asp 800-647-6100

[85] Goldstat R, Briganti E, Tran J, Wolfe R, Davis SR. Transdermal testosterone therapy improves well-being, mood, and sexual function in premenopausal women. *Menopause. 2003 Sep-Oct: 10(5):390-8.*

[86] Xie B, Tsao SW, Wong YC. Sex hormone-induced mammary carcinogenesis in the female Noble rats: expression of bcl-2 and bax in hormonal mammary carcinogenesis. *Breast Cancer Res Treat. 2000 May;61(1):45-57.*

[87] Xie B, Tsao SW, Wong YC. Sex hormone-induced mammary carcinogenesis in female Noble rats: expression of TGF-beta1 and its receptors, TGF-alpha, and EGF-R in mammary carcinogenesis. *Breast Cancer Res Treat. 1999 Dec;58(3):227-39.*

[88] Ness RB, Albano JD, McTiernan A, Cauley JA. Influence of estrogen plus testosterone supplementation on breast cancer. *Arch Intern Med. 2009 Jan12;169(1):41-6.*

[89] Bitzer J, Kenemans P, Mueck AO; FSD education Group. Breast cancer risk in postmenopausal women using testosterone in combination with hormone replacement therapy. *Maturitas. 2008 Mar 20;59(3):209-18.*

[90] Notelovitz M. Androgen effects on bone and muscle. *Fertil Steril. 2002 Apr;77 Suppl 4:S34-41.*

[91] Korenman SG, Morley JE, Mooradian AD, Davis SS, Kaiser FE, Silver AJ, Viosca SP, Garza D. Secondary hypogonadism in older men: its relation to impotence. *J Clin Endocrinol Metab. 1990 Oct;71(4):963-9.*

[92] Travison TG, Araujo AB, O'Donnell AB, Kupelian V, McKinlay JB. A population-level decline in serum testosterone levels in American men. *J Clin Endocrinol Metab. 2007 Jan;92(1):196-202.*

[93] Shores MM, Matsumoto AM, Sloan KL, Kivlahan DR. Low serum testosterone and mortality in male veterans. *Arch Intern Med. 2006 Aug 14;166(15):1660-5.*

[94] Raynaud, JP. Prostate cancer risk in testosterone-treated men. *J Steroid Biochem Mol Biol. 2006 Dec;102(1-5):261-6.*

[95] Sawada N, Iwasaki M, Inoue M, Sasazuki S, Yamaji T, Shimazu T, Tsugane S; for the Japan Public Health Center-based Prospective Study Group. Plasma testosterone and sex hormone-binding globulin concentrations and the risk of prostate cancer among Japanese men: A nested case-control study. *Cancer Sci. 2010 Dec;101(12):2652-2657.*

[96] Morgentaler A. Testosterone and prostate cancer: an historical perspective on a modern myth. *Eur Urol. 2006 Nov;50(5):935-9.*

[97] Mustafa A, Nyberg F, Mustafa M, Bakhiet M, Mustafa E, Winblad B, Adem A. Growth hormone stimulates production of interferon-gamma by human peripheral mononuclear cells. *Horm Res. 1997;48(1):11-5.*

[98] Wright YL. *Secrets about Bioidentical Hormones to Lose Fat and Prevent Cancer, Heart Disease, Menopause, and Andropause, by Optimizing Adrenals, Thyroid, Estrogen, Progesterone, Testosterone, and Growth Hormone!* Lulu.com. December 18, 2010. p. 61.

[99] Wright YL. *Secrets about Bioidentical Hormones to Lose Fat and Prevent Cancer, Heart Disease, Menopause, and Andropause, by Optimizing Adrenals, Thyroid, Estrogen, Progesterone, Testosterone, and Growth Hormone!* Lulu.com. December 18, 2010. p. 27.

[100] Malkin CJ, Pugh PJ, Jones RD, Kapoor D, Channer KS, Jones TH. The effect of testosterone replacement on endogenous inflammatory cytokines and lipid profiles in hypogonadal men. *J Clin Endocrinol Metab. 2004 Jul;89(7):33118-8.*

[101] Channer KS, Jones TH. Cardiovascular effects of testosterone: implications of the "male menopause"? *Heart. 2003 Feb;89(2):121-2.*

[102] English KM, Steeds RP, Jones TH, Diver MJ, Channer KS. Low-dose transdermal testosterone therapy improves angina threshold in men with chronic stable angina: A randomized, double-blind, placebo-controlled study. *Circulation 2000. Oct 17; 102(16):1906-11.*

[103] Malkin CJ, Pugh PJ, Morris PD, Kerry KE, Jones RD, Jones TH, Channer KS. Testosterone replacement in hypogonadal men with angina improves ischaemic threshold and quality of life. *Heart. 2004 Aug;90(8):871-6.*

[104] Rosano GM, Leonardo F, Pagnotta P, Pelliccia F, Panina G, Cerquetani E, della Monica PL, Bonfigli B, Volpe M, Chierchia SL. Acute anti-ischemic effect of testosterone in men with coronary artery disease. *Circulation 1999 Apr 6;99(13):1666-70.*

[105] Webb CM, McNeill JG, Hayward CS, de Zeigler D, Collins P. Effects of testosterone on coronary vasomotor regulation in men with coronary heart disease. *Circulation. 1999 Oct 19;100(16):1690-6.*

[106] Khaw KT, Barrett-Connor E. Blood pressure and endogenous testosterone in men: an inverse relationship. *J Hypertens. 1988 Apr;6(4):329-32.*

[107] Boyanov MA, Boneva Z, Christov VG. Testosterone supplementation in men with type 2 diabetes, visceral obesity and partial androgen deficiency. *Aging Male. 2003 Mar; 6(1):1-7.*

[108] Cooper MA, Ritchie EC. Testosterone replacement therapy for anxiety. *Am J Psychiatry. 2000 Nov;157(11):1884.*

[109] Bhasin S. The dose-dependent effects of testosterone on sexual function and on muscle mass and function. *Mayo Clin Proc. 2000 Jan;75 Suppl:S70-5.*

[110] Roddam AW, Allen NE, Appleby P, Key TJ. Endogenous Hormones and Prostate Cancer Collaborative Group. Endogenous Sex Hormones and Prostate Cancer: A Collaborative Analysis of 18 Prospective Studies. *J Natl Cancer Inst. 2008 Feb 6;100(3):170-83.*

[111] Gould DC. and Kirby RS. Testosterone replacement therapy for late onset hypogonadism: what is the risk of inducing prostate cancer? *Prostate Cancer Prostatic Dis. 2006; 9(1):14-8.*

[112] Feneley MR, Carruthers ME. PSA monitoring during testosterone replacement therapy: low long-term risk of prostate cancer with improved opportunity for cure. *Andrologia 2004; 36:212.*

[113] Morgentaler A. Guideline for male testosterone therapy: a clinician's perspective. *J Clin Endocrinol Metab. 2007 Feb;92(2):416-7.*

[114] Marks LS, Mazer NA, Mostaghel E, Hess DL, Dorey FJ, Epstein JI, Veltri RW, Makarov DV, Partin AW, Bostwick DG, Macairan ML, Nelson PS. Effect of testosterone replacement therapy on prostate tissue in men with late-onset hypogonadism: a randomized controlled trial. *JAMA. 2006 Nov 15;296(19):2351-61.*

[115] Moffat SD, Resnick SM. Long-term measures of free testosterone predict regional cerebral blood flow patterns in elderly men. *Neurobiol Aging. 2007 Jun;28(6):914-20.*

[116] Gouras GK, Xu H, Gross RS, Greenfield JP, Hai B, Wang R, Greengard P. Testosterone reduces neuronal secretion of beta amyloid peptides. *Proc Natl Acad Sci U S A 2000 Feb 1;97(3):1202-5.*

[117] Burris AS, Banks SM, Carter CS, Davidson JM, Sherins RJ. A long-term, prospective study of the physiologic and behavioral effects of hormone replacement in untreated hypogonadal men. *J Androl 1992 Jul-Aug; 13(4)297-304.*

[118] Tan RS, Pu SJ. A pilot study on the effects of testosterone in hypogonadal aging male

patients with Alzheimer's disease. *Aging Male. 3003 Mar;6(1):13-7.*

[119] Alexander GM, Swerdloff RS, Wang C, Davidson T, McDonald V, Steiner B, Hines M. Androgen-behavior correlations in hypogonadal men and eugonadal men. *II. Cognitive abilities. Horm Behav. 1998 Apr;33(2):85-94.*

[120] Barrett-Connor E, Goodman-Gruen D, Patay B. Endogenous sex hormones and cognitive function in older men. *J Clin Endocrinol Metab 1999 Oct; 84(10):3681-5.*

[121] Muniyappa R, Sorkin JD, Veldhuis JD, Harman SM, Münzer T, Bhasin S, Blackman MR. Long-term testosterone supplementation augments overnight growth hormone secretion in healthy older men. *Am J Physiol Endocrinol Metab. 2007 Sep;293(3):E769-75.*

[122] Caretta N, Ferlin A, Palego PF, Foresta C. Erectile dysfunction in aging men: testosterone role in therapeutic protocols. *J Endocrinol Invest. 2005;28(11 Suppl Proceedings):108-11.*

[123] Foresta C, Caretta N, Lana A, De Toni L, Biagioli A, Ferlin A, Garolla A. Reduced number of circulating Endothelial Progenitor Cells in hypogonadal men. *Journal of Clinical Endocrinology and Metabolism 91(11)4599-4602.*

[124] Heinonen OP, Albanes D, Virtamo J, Taylor PR, Huttunen JK, Hartman AM, Haapakoski J, Malila N, Rautalahti M, Ripatti S, Mäenpää H, Teerenhovi L, Koss L, Virolainen M, Edwards BK. Prostate cancer and supplementation with alpha-tocopherol and beta-carotene: incidence and mortality in a controlled trial. *J Natl Cancer Inst. 1998 Mar 18;90(6):440-6.*

[125] Wright YL. *Secrets about Bioidentical Hormones to Lose Fat and Prevent Cancer, Heart Disease, Menopause, and Andropause, by Optimizing Adrenals, Thyroid, Estrogen, Progesterone, Testosterone, and Growth Hormone!* Lulu.com. December 18, 2010. p. 38.

[126] Jeng YJ, Watson CS. Combinations of Physiologic Estrogens with Xenoestrogens Alter ERK Phosphorylation Profiles in Rat Pituitary Cells. *Environ Health Perspect. 2010 Sep 22.*

[127] Darbre PD, Charles AK. Environmental oestrogens and breast cancer: evidence for combined involvement of dietary, household and cosmetic xenoestrogens. *Anticancer Res. 2010 Mar; 30(3):815-27.*

[128] Dallinga JW, Moonen EJ, Dumoulin JC, Evers JL, Geraedts JP, Kleinjans JC. Decreased human semen quality and organochlorine compounds in blood. *Hum Reprod. 2002 Aug;17(8):1973-9.*

[129] Ellison PT, Panter-Brick C, Lipson SF, O'Rourke MT. The ecological context of human ovarian function. *Hum Reprod. 1993 Dec;8(12):2248-58.*

[130] Wetherill YB, Fisher NL, Staubach A, Danielsen M, de Vere White RW, Knudsen KE. Xenoestrogen action in prostate cancer: pleiotropic effects dependent on androgen receptor status. *Cancer Res. 2005 Jan 1;65(1):54-65.*

[131] Maffini MV, Rubin BS, Sonnenschein C, Soto AM. Endocrine disruptors and reproductive health: the case of bisphenol-A. *Mol Cell Endocrinol. 2006 Jul 25;254 255:179-86.*

[132] Skinner MK, Manikkam M, Guerrero-Bosagna C. Epigenetic Transgenerational ACTIONS OF ENDOCRINE DISRUPTORS. *Reprod Toxicol. 2010 Nov 2.*

[133] Wagner M, Oehlmann J. Endocrine disruptors in bottled mineral water: Estrogenic activity in the E-Screen. J *Steroid Biochem Mol Biol. 2010 Nov 1.*

[134] Ruzzin J, Petersen R, Meugnier E, Madsen L, Lock EJ, Lillefosse H, Ma T, Pesenti S, Sonne SB, Marstrand TT, Malde MK, Du ZY, Chavey C, Fajas L, Lundebye AK, Brand CL, Vidal H, Kristiansen K, Frøyland L. Persistent organic pollutant exposure leads to insulin resistance syndrome. *Environ Health Perspect. 2010 Apr;118(4):465-71.*

[135] Ferrucci LM, Sinha R, Ward MH, Graubard BI, Hollenbeck AR, Kilfoy BA, Schatzkin A, Michaud DS, Cross AJ. Meat and components of meat and the risk of bladder cancer in the NIH-AARP Diet and Health Study. *Cancer. 2010 Sep 15;116(18):4345-53.*

[136] Alexander JC. Chemical and biological properties related to toxicity of heated fats. *J Toxicol Environ Health. 1981 Jan;7(1):125-38.*

[137] Castro-Martínez MG, Bolado-García VE, Landa-Anell MV, Liceaga-Cravioto MG, Soto-González J, López-Alvarenga JC. [Dietary trans fatty acids and its metabolic implications].

Gac Med Mex. 2010 Jul-Aug;146(4):281-8. Spanish.

[138] Bustnes JO, Lie E, Herzke D, Dempster T, Bjørn PA, Nygård T, Uglem I. Salmon Farms as a Source of Organohalogenated Contaminants in Wild Fish. *Environ Sci Technol. 2010 Nov 15;44(22):8736-8743.*

[139] Nierenberg D. Rethinking the global meat industry. *State of the World 2006; Worldwatch Institute:p.26.*

[140] Reece RL, Barr DA, Forsyth WM, Scott PC. Investigations of toxicity episodes involving chemotherapeutic agents in Victorian poultry and pigeons. *Avian Dis.1985 Oct-Dec;29(4):1239-51.*

[141] Gutowska I, Baranowska-Bosiacka I, Baśkiewicz M, Milo B, Siennicka A, Marchlewicz M, Wiszniewska B, Machaliński B, Stachowska E. Fluoride as a pro-inflammatory factor and inhibitor of ATP bioavailability in differentiated human THP1 monocytic cells. *Toxicol Lett. 2010 Jul 1;196(2):74-9.*

[142] Focke F, Schuermann D, Kuster N, Schär P (November 2009). DNA fragmentation in human fibroblasts under extremely low frequency electromagnetic field exposure. *Mutation Research 683* (1-2): 74–83.

[143] Ros E, Tapsell LC, Sabaté J. Nuts and berries for heart health. *Curr Atheroscler Rep. 2010 Nov;12(6):397-406.*

[144] Weaver CM, Martin BR, Story JA, Hutchinson I, Sanders L. Novel Fibers Increase Bone Calcium Content and Strength beyond Efficiency of Large Intestine Fermentation. *J Agric Food Chem. 2010 Aug 2.*

[145] Bidoli E, Pelucchi C, Zucchetto A, Negri E, Dal Maso L, Polesel J, Montella M, Franceschi S, Serraino D, La Vecchia C, Talamini R. Fiber intake and endometrial cancer risk. *Acta Oncol. 2010 May;49(4):441-6.*

[146] Fork FT, Ekberg O, Nilsson G, Rerup C, Skinhøj A. Colon cleansing regimens. A clinical study in 1200 patients. *Gastrointest Radiol. 1982;7(4):383-9.*

[147] Genuis SJ, Birkholz D, Ralitsch M, Thibault N. Human detoxification of perfluorinated compounds. *Public Health. 2010 Jul;124(7):367-75.*

[148] Krop J. Chemical sensitivity after intoxication at work with solvents: response to sauna therapy. *J Altern Complement Med. 1998 Spring;4(1):77-86.*

[149] Gerson M. The cure of advanced cancer by diet therapy: a summary of 30 years of clinical experimentation. *Physiol Chem Phys. 1978;10(5):449-64.*

[150] Lam LK, Sparnins VL, Wattenberg LW. Effects of derivatives of kahweol and cafestol on the activity of glutathione S-transferase in mice. *J Med Chem. 1987 Aug;30(8):1399-403.*

[151] Uchikawa T, Yasutake A, Kumamoto Y, Maruyama I, Kumamoto S, Ando Y. The influence of Parachlorella beyerinckii CK-5 on the absorption and excretion of methylmercury (MeHg) in mice. *J Toxicol Sci. 2010;35(1):101-5.*

[152] Pore RS. Detoxification of chlordecone poisoned rats with chlorella and chlorella derived sporopollenin. *Drug Chem Toxicol. 1984;7(1):57-71.*

[153] Huang Z, Li L, Huang G, Yan Q, Shi B, Xu X. Growth-inhibitory and metal-binding proteins in Chlorella vulgaris exposed to cadmium or zinc. *Aquat Toxicol. 2009 Jan 18;91(1):54-61.*

[154] Frisardi V, Solfrizzi V, Capurso C, Kehoe PG, Imbimbo BP, Santamato A, Dellegrazie F, Seripa D, Pilotto A, Capurso A, Panza F. Aluminum in the diet and Alzheimer's disease: from current epidemiology to possible disease-modifying treatment. *J Alzheimers Dis. 2010;20(1):17-30.*

[155] Selye H. *The Stress of Life.* New York, Toronto, London: McGraw-Hill Book Company, 1956.

[156] Wright YL. *Secrets about Bioidentical Hormones to Lose Fat and Prevent Cancer, Heart Disease, Menopause, and Andropause, by Optimizing Adrenals, Thyroid, Estrogen, Progesterone, Testosterone, and Growth Hormone!* Lulu.com. December 18, 2010. p. 40.

[157] Wright YL. *Secrets about Bioidentical Hormones to Lose Fat and Prevent Cancer, Heart Disease, Menopause, and Andropause, by Optimizing Adrenals, Thyroid, Estrogen,*

Progesterone, Testosterone, and Growth Hormone! Lulu.com. December 18, 2010. p. 43.

[158] Epel E, Lapidus R, McEwen B, Brownell K. Stress may add bite to appetite in women: a laboratory study of stress-induced cortisol and eating behavior. *Psychoneuroendocrinology 2001 Jan;26(1):37-49*

[159] Wright YL. *Secrets about Bioidentical Hormones to Lose Fat and Prevent Cancer, Heart Disease, Menopause, and Andropause, by Optimizing Adrenals, Thyroid, Estrogen, Progesterone, Testosterone, and Growth Hormone!* Lulu.com. December 18, 2010. p. 44.

[160] Wright YL. *Secrets about Bioidentical Hormones to Lose Fat and Prevent Cancer, Heart Disease, Menopause, and Andropause, by Optimizing Adrenals, Thyroid, Estrogen, Progesterone, Testosterone, and Growth Hormone!* Lulu.com. December 18, 2010. p. 87.

[161] http://somaticexperiencing.com

[162] http://upledger.com   (800) 233-5880

[163] http://www.emdr.com/index.htm (831) 761-1040

[164] http://www.findyourpathhome.com (303) 775-3431

[165] Rossouw JE, Anderson GL, Prentice RL, LaCroix AZ, Kooperberg C, Stefanick ML, Jackson RD, Beresford SA, Howard BV, Johnson KC, Kotchen JM, Ockene J; Writing Group for the Women's Health Initiative Investigators. Risks and benefits of estrogen plus progestin in healthy postmenopausal women: principal results From the Women's Health Initiative randomized controlled trial. *JAMA. 2002 Jul 17;288(3):321-33.*

[166] Chlebowski RT, Kuller LH, Prentice RL, Stefanick ML, Manson JE, Gass M, Aragaki AK, Ockene JK, Lane DS, Sarto GE, Rajkovic A, Schenken R, Hendrix SL, Ravdin PM, Rohan TE, Yasmeen S, Anderson G; WHI Investigators. Breast cancer after use of estrogen plus progestin in postmenopausal women. *N Engl J Med. 2009 Feb 5;360(6):573-87.*

[167] Fournier A, Berrino F, Riboli E, Avenel V, Clavel-Chapelon F. Breast cancer risk in relation to different types of hormone replacement therapy in the E3N-EPIC cohort. *Int J Cancer. 2005 Apr 10; 114(3):448-54.*

[168] Lippert TH, Mueck AO, Seeger H. Is the use of conjugated equine oestrogens in hormone replacement therapy still appropriate? *Chem Res Toxicol. 1999 Feb;12(2):204-13.*

[169] http://www.worldhealth.net/pages/directory/   888-997-0112

[170] http://www.acamnet.org/ 800-532-3688

[171] Wright YL. *Secrets about Bioidentical Hormones to Lose Fat and Prevent Cancer, Heart Disease, Menopause, and Andropause, by Optimizing Adrenals, Thyroid, Estrogen, Progesterone, Testosterone, and Growth Hormone!* Lulu.com. December 18, 2010. p. 13.

[172] Wright YL. *Secrets about Bioidentical Hormones to Lose Fat and Prevent Cancer, Heart Disease, Menopause, and Andropause, by Optimizing Adrenals, Thyroid, Estrogen, Progesterone, Testosterone, and Growth Hormone!* Lulu.com. December 18, 2010. p. 40.

[173] Wright YL. *Secrets about Bioidentical Hormones to Lose Fat and Prevent Cancer, Heart Disease, Menopause, and Andropause, by Optimizing Adrenals, Thyroid, Estrogen, Progesterone, Testosterone, and Growth Hormone!* Lulu.com. December 18, 2010. p. 78.

[174] Wright YL. *Secrets about Bioidentical Hormones to Lose Fat and Prevent Cancer, Heart Disease, Menopause, and Andropause, by Optimizing Adrenals, Thyroid, Estrogen, Progesterone, Testosterone, and Growth Hormone!* Lulu.com. December 18, 2010. p. 78.

Index